Difficult Psychiatric Consultations

Sergio V. Delgado • Jeffrey R. Strawn

Difficult Psychiatric Consultations

An Integrated Approach

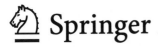 Springer

Sergio V. Delgado
Department of Psychiatry
  and Child Psychiatry
Cincinnati Children's Hospital
  Medical Center
Cincinnati
Ohio, USA

Jeffrey R. Strawn
Department of Psychiatry
  and Behavioral Neuroscience
University of Cincinnati
Cincinnati
Ohio, USA

ISBN 978-3-642-39551-2   ISBN 978-3-642-39552-9 (eBook)
DOI 10.1007/978-3-642-39552-9
Springer Heidelberg New York Dordrecht London

Library of Congress Control Number: 2013953921

Printed on acid-free paper

Springer is part of Springer Science+Business Media (www.springer.com)

To Michelle Alexandra and Erin.
—SVD

To Lara Suzanne and my parents.
—JRS

Preface

This book is written with several audiences and several aims in mind. First, we aim to expand the psychiatric consultation literature and to present an effective, collaborative approach to working with the complex or "difficult psychiatric consultations." Second, we aim to integrate what have been historically seen as competing psychological theories into a useful and effective approach to psychiatric consultation involving patients, families, and treatment teams that present with competing agendas. Third, we aim to guide experienced clinicians, psychiatric residents, clinical fellows, as well as clinical psychologists to use a multi-dimensional approach with difficult clinical consultations. Herein, we provide relevant cases that allow the reader to be in the mind of the psychiatric consultant and also include tables that allow for a practical approach to review relevant information to be used in tailoring the interventions needed. We are aware that, despite the effectiveness of these psychodynamic and family-based approaches to the patient, ground is rapidly being lost to "*DSM*-only" focused approaches and more limited biologic and psychopharmacologic interventions.

We also recognize that, as with any approach, there will be skeptics. Among the arguments that may be levied against this strategy is that multiple theoretically diverse approaches cannot be fully integrated. However, we would argue that these seemingly disparate theories are already integrated within our difficult clinical consultations, in that the issues related to family systems, attachment styles, relational processes, and cognition are part and parcel of everyday consultative work. Second, the argument may be made that our approach involves closeness with the patient, the family, and the treatment team and that this closeness could compromise "true objectivity." Certainly however, we now recognize—based on contributions from attachment theory and intersubjectivity—that "true objectivity" is a relative myth. What a treatment team may view as an enmeshed family in fact may be functioning in a psychologically and culturally appropriate way which facilitates compliance by the patient. Third, some practitioners may be concerned that this approach would be prohibitive because of the time involvement. Here, we would note that in difficult clinical consultations, the mild increase in time involvement is justified as cases with high family, patient, and treatment-team conflict tend to have greater adverse outcomes, longer hospitalizations, and a greater likelihood of medical–legal sequelae. Thus, we would argue that this approach, while somewhat more time-intensive, is more cost-effective.

The decision to write this book originated in the fall of 2011 when members of the American Academy of Child and Adolescent Psychiatry Committees on Psychotherapy, Family, and Ethics were asked to develop a collaborative program to integrate psychotherapeutic, family systems, and ethical aspects of "difficult" cases. After some discussion, it became apparent that the consulting psychiatrist working with "difficult" consultations in adults was often encumbered by these same issues. We quickly realized that clinicians had an urgent need for a practical and clinically-relevant approach to integrate these clinical perspectives with regard to psychodynamic thinking, family systems, and ethical aspects of the cases.

We hope that this book provides the *student*, in the broader sense of the term, with a clear, relevant, and practical approach to the difficult psychiatric consultation. Ultimately, this book will have day-to-day clinical relevance to the practicing psychiatrist. Herein, we emphasize the value of collaboration in the consultation process and describe the ways in which a well-aligned, multidisciplinary treatment team can provide a sense of safety, compassion, and understanding for the patient and his family. However, we also provide examples of the misaligned treatment team and strategies to prevent treatment sabotage. The intimate and complex work with a difficult psychiatric consultation is essential to the personal and professional growth of a psychiatrist. The capacity to tolerate strong affects and integrate varied perspectives provides a sense of security and comfort to the distressed patient or family by creating what psychoanalyst and pediatrician Donald Winnicot, M.D., termed a "holding environment." Finally, we hope that the seasoned clinician may be able to use this book as a practical guide to help his or her trainees to embark on more in-depth discussions of psychodynamic, family systems, cultural, and ethical aspects of patients' illnesses, as the attention to these topics has waned over the last several decades.

Cincinnati, OH   Sergio V. Delgado
                                                                      Jeffrey R. Strawn

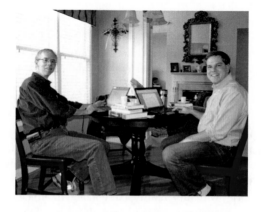

Acknowledgments

We would like to express our heartfelt gratitude to our patients, who unknowingly contributed to this book in remarkable ways, providing the clinical material and keeping us on our toes when working with them. We also wish to thank our mentors and teachers, who provided the foundation for our appreciation of the multiple theories and complexities that must be considered if we are to understand our patients and their families. Additionally, we are indebted to our students, who helped us appreciate the pressures of trying to "fit in" as one learns about psychodynamic and family systems theories, and we especially thank those students who courageously challenged us (and our theoretical approaches) when needed.

We want to express our warm thanks to Corinna Schaefer, associate editor, clinical medicine for Springer Publishing. We were surprised, honored, and scared to death when she asked if we would write this book. Her steadfast support has provided the energy behind these pages. Importantly, Corinna believed in us and supported this project in spite of the many changes we made. Also, we wish to thank Nicola Mason for her fantastic editorial assistance, her attention to detail, and her ability to make clearer our sometimes muddled sentiments with her masterful use of the written word and grammatical prowess.

We are grateful to our fellow AACAP members, Mary Cook, M.D., Basil Bernstein, M.D., and Heather Adams, M.D., for their guidance and thoughtful comments as we prepared our presentation "What's your angle? Bringing clarity to complex clinical presentations, integrating psychodynamic, family systems, medico-legal, and ethical lenses," which provided the inspiration for this work. We are deeply indebted to those who read our manuscript and were kind enough to be "not so kind" in pointing out what we had missed or did not get right. Kirby Pope, M.D., our close friend who read the first draft of this manuscript, was gentle in sharing comments that helped shape the flow of the content, as was our colleague Elizabeth Burstein, M.S.W., who also read selected chapters and was not shy in providing constructive criticism. We also express our gratitude to Michael Sorter, M.D., who kindly supported our work on this project. To all, we say thank you!

I am indebted to Erin, my true better half, who provided the warmth that kept me from giving up, provided the useful "unedited" critiques needed to improve the readability of this book, and was instrumental in helping the authors keep their eyes on the project as there were plenty of times we would have preferred to quit. Finally, I want to thank my friend and co-author Jeff, who tolerated my Hispanic and "old school" approach to the material and was able to maintain our close friendship despite our not-so-subtle disagreements.

—SVD

This work would not have been possible without the loving support of my wife, Lara, who from the beginning helped me to balance our life with the writing of this book, although she may still not agree that we reached equilibrium. Also, I thank my parents, my first teachers of attachment theory, who provided the early developmental experiences that made the writing of this book possible. Finally, I thank my friend and co-author, Sergio, whose (sometimes) gentle encouragement of my writing and always-present enthusiasm were the driving force for *Difficult Psychiatric Consultations*: *An Integrated Approach*.

—JRS

Contents

Introduction

There's no such thing as a baby
—Donald W. Winnicott (1896–1971)

Over 60 years ago, the English pediatrician and psychoanalyst Donald W. Winnicott (1896–1971) astutely observed: "There's no such thing as a baby" (Winnicott 1964/1947). Today, most psychiatrists are keenly aware that there's no such thing as a "patient"; that is, a patient exists inside an environment that includes their families, the treating physicians, treatment teams, subspecialty consultants, and other clinical providers. In turn, a patient's interactions with these groups are heavily influenced by their prior experiences, cognitive styles, attachment patterns, temperaments, and most importantly, their cultural backgrounds. Frequently, for most of those in need of aid, treatment is effectively provided and received, and recovery ensues. However, when treatment does not go according to plan, the parties involved can experience anxieties that lead to unexpected negative outcomes. If the patient's treatment becomes derailed due to their personality or to cognitive problems, the treatment team begins to view the patient as "noncompliant" or "difficult," and they request a psychiatric consultation. When the patient's treatment becomes thwarted by family factors, psychiatrists are also asked to provide insight. These consultations may result in recommendations regarding psychopharmacologic strategies for various neuropsychiatric disorders (e.g., delirium, depression secondary to α-interferon therapy, postpartum psychosis) or the clarifying of psychiatric diagnoses. Sometimes, however, clinical consultations are much more complex and fraught—"difficult clinical consultations"—requiring an integrated effort that combines the careful assessment of the patient from a multidimensional perspective (psychodynamic, family, and ethical) with an informed strategy for the treatment team and the patient's family. In *Difficult Psychiatric Consultations: An Integrated Approach*, we will describe effective approaches to difficult psychiatric consultations and in doing so will comprehensively discuss issues and impediments related to the patient, the family, and the treatment team. In addition, we'll explore the ethical and cultural aspects of managing these "difficult consultations." Our goal in presenting this systematic

S.V. Delgado and J.R. Strawn, *Difficult Psychiatric Consultations*,
DOI 10.1007/978-3-642-39552-9_1, © Springer-Verlag Berlin Heidelberg 2014

approach is to facilitate the psychiatric consultant's work within the larger healthcare system and to provide reliable and usable tools for the consultant who works with complex patients and their treatment teams.

1.1   From Psychiatric Consultation to "Psychosomatic Medicine"

Psychiatric consultation has evolved over the last half century. What is now known as "psychosomatic medicine" began in the early 1940s and, during these early years, was often referred to as "consultation-liaison" psychiatry. A reflection of the early goals within the field, consultation-liaison psychiatry involved providing assistance to medically-oriented physicians in managing the psychiatric problems of the medically ill population in hospital settings and also in negotiating conflicts surrounding emotionally charged decisions or aspects of care. Later, consultation-liaison psychiatry formally became a subspecialty that incorporated clinical practice, teaching, and research at the borderland of psychiatry and medicine (Hunter et al. 2007; Lipowski 1983). Today, this subspecialty is referred to as psychosomatic medicine, and was formally recognized by the American Psychiatric Association in 2004 (Gitlin et al. 2004). Though psychosomatic medicine is well situated as a psychiatric subspecialty, the term itself has not become standard in medical settings, and the use of "consultation-liaison psychiatry" remains favored and will be used throughout this book. As McIntyre (2002) aptly stated, "The name of this subspecialty has been debated for years, and the choice of the name 'psychosomatic medicine' will not end the discussion." He concludes: "Consultation-liaison has indeed made, and continues to make, major contributions to the practice of medicine and the education of physicians. Whatever its name, its best days lie ahead" (McIntyre 2002).

Consultation-liaison psychiatry embodies the bio-psycho-social treatment (Engel 1977, 1980) approach more than perhaps any other subspecialty. Recently, the bio-psycho-social model has come to represent the "progressive unification of the medical and behavioral sciences, including psychiatry, in a search for etiological and preventive factors in human health and disease" and underscores the importance of seeing patients as "'united, bio-psycho-social persons' rather than as 'biomedical persons' divorced from their psychological and social dimensions" (Dowling 2005). However, some have argued that this model poses demands on physicians that interfere with their clinical activities, and that bio-psycho-social issues are best addressed by consultation-liaison psychiatry. The financial implications of the care provided by physicians were also considered a relevant factor that limited its use. Nonetheless, this model, in George Engel's words, "motivates the physician to become more informed and skillful in psychosocial areas, disciplines now seen as alien and remote unit by those who intuitively recognize their importance. . . . [It] serves to counteract the wasteful reductionist pursuit of what often prove to be trivial rather than crucial determinants of illness. The bio-psycho-social physician is expected to have working knowledge of the principles, language, and basic facts of each of the relevant discipline, he is not expected to be an expert in all" (Engel 1980). Encouraging involvement with psychiatric services, the bio-psycho-social model forwards the precept that only in addressing the psychological and social factors (e.g., cultural background and family) can the patient be effectively treated.

1.2   The Psychiatric Consultant's "Job Description"

The psychiatric consultant practicing in today's busy medical center has numerous responsibilities and collaborates with many members of the medical staff, midlevel providers, and nurses, as well as with social workers and case managers. Traditionally, the consultant's job was to determine the psychiatric diagnosis, provide recommendations regarding psychopharmacologic management, assist with conflict negotiation, distinguish the psychiatric from the psychosocial, and help determine the patient's decision-making capacity; "be familiar with the routines of the medical/surgical environment and knowledgeable about medical and surgical illness. . .and aware of the effects that illness and drugs have on behavior, especially when they contribute to or confound the diagnosis or treatment [of the "medical-psychiatric" patient]" (Bronheim et al. 1998). The modern psychiatric consultant is additionally and importantly charged with providing a framework that the treatment team can use to promote a bio-psycho-social model, a framework that both guides their interventions and enhances the patient's medical or psychological treatment. The effective consultant helps to bridge the patient's subjective, illness-related perceptions, and the expertise of the treatment team that designs the necessary therapeutic interventions for him or her. The psychiatrist is also tasked with creating a psychological space that facilitates open communication, enabling the patient to convey distress and the treatment team to reassure the patient that its efforts are aimed at improving the medical outcome. When a diagnosis of a medical or psychiatric illness is given—whether or not the condition is short-term or chronic—the patient's sense of invincibility is shattered, and the treatment team's goal is to engender a sense of hopefulness, offering strategies and teaching coping skills that the patient can employ to attain, as closely as possible, the level of functioning they had before the diagnosis.

1.3   The Psychiatric Resident Consultant's "Job Description"

In academic medical centers with active psychiatric residency and fellowship programs, many of the functions described above may be initially performed by a resident or fellow, albeit with direct supervision by a psychiatrist. We recognize that with consultations provided by a resident or fellow, the trainee has a unique responsibility to obtain guidance from the faculty psychiatric consultant, and that the faculty member has ultimate responsibility for the patient's consultation (Streltzer and Hoyle 2007; Wei et al. 2011). In teaching trainees consultation psychiatry, the approach described in this book will facilitate active learning and successful integration of multiple theoretical approaches. As residents have been shown to prefer an "eclectic" approach to consultation, "integrating techniques from a variety of modalities rather than a comprehensive or specific modality" (Hunter et al. 2007), the faculty psychiatric consultant can best teach the resident in using a developmental timeline, informed by the bio-psycho-social model. As Gabbard and Kay (2001) have noted, "residents should be taught that the biopsychosocial model is crucial in every clinical setting, including hospital treatment, consultation-liaison work, medication management, and managed care."

1.4   Limitations of Psychosomatic Medicine

In the recent psychosomatic-medicine literature, the main focus has been on the consequences of the patient's reaction to his or her condition and on the co-morbidities that occur with medical illness (Levenson 2002). Little attention has been given to the reaction of the patient's family, including siblings, and to the ways the treatment team interacts with its patients as well as the family (Kazak 2001; Williams 1997). Treatment-team members may deliberately create emotional distance so as to make appropriate decisions without being affected or influenced by the patient's anxieties. It is important to recognize, however, that these team members are also human participants, and that they can use their empathy to bolster the patient's strengths rather than withdraw and allow his or her anxiety to intensify. In this text, the processes surrounding the network of influences on the patient will be extensively reviewed and demystified, and we will offer examples of tactical interventions for the psychiatric consultant to use in working through "difficult consultations" with "difficult patients" as well as with the treatment teams themselves.

Interestingly, the role of the "psychopharmacologist" consultant has received increased attention in contemporary discussions of consultation models (Kontos et al. 2006). Some psychopharmacologists choose to focus on the accuracy of the diagnosis with the use of structured clinical interviews of the patient, aided by rating scales (e.g., Hamilton Anxiety Rating Scale (Hamilton 1959), Hamilton Depression Rating Scale (Hamilton 1960), Delirium Rating Scale, and Inventory of Depressive Symptoms (Rush et al. 1996)). Though this approach may at times be preferred by those wishing to *strictly* adhere to evidence-based medicine—i.e., wishing to choose the intervention specifically addressing *Diagnostic and Statistical Manual of Mental Disorders 5th Edition* (*DSM-5*, APA 2013) "primary diagnosis"—by not considering how the patient's personality characteristics contribute to outcome, the treatment team may lose its opportunity to establish a supportive partnership with the patient and family that would encourage both compliance and adherence to the treatment plan. Accordingly, we advocate that even the psychopharmacologist would be better served by understanding the interrelations among the treatment-team members, the patient, and his or her family, as well as by attending to constitutional aspects of the patient—cognitive flexibility, temperament, psychological defenses, etc.—that may complicate or facilitate successful psychopharmacologic interventions.

1.5 How to Use This Book

This book is written with several audiences and several goals in mind. First, we aim to expand the psychiatric-consultation literature and to present an effective collaborative method of working with complex or difficult clinical consultations. Second, we seek to integrate what have been historically seen as competing psychological theories while addressing psychiatric consultation involving patients, families, and treatment teams that present with competing agendas. Third, we aim to guide experienced clinicians, psychiatric residents, and clinical fellows, as well as clinical psychologists, toward using a multidimensional approach with complex psychiatric consultations (Fig. 1.1).

Herein, we provide relevant cases that allow the reader to be on the shoulder of the psychiatric consultant and that also include tables for efficient review relevant information while tailoring the interventions needed.

Despite the advantages of the approach we are advocating here, we recognize that, as with any approach, there will be skeptics. Among the arguments that may be levied against our strategy is that multiple theoretically diverse approaches cannot be fully integrated. We would argue, however, that these seemingly disparate theories are already integrated within our difficult consultations, in that the issues related to family systems, attachment styles, relational processes, and cognition are part and parcel of everyday consultative work. The argument may also be made that our methods invite closeness with the patient, the family, and the treatment team, and that this intimacy could compromise "true objectivity"—though surely, based on contributions from attachment theory and intersubjectivity, we must recognize that "true objectivity" is a relative myth. What a treatment team might view as an enmeshed family may be in fact functioning in a psychologically and culturally appropriate manner that facilitates compliance by the patient, as will be described in Chap. 7. To practitioners concerned that this approach will require a prohibitive amount of time, we would note that in difficult consultations, the mild increase in time commitment is justified, as cases with high family, patient, and treatment-team conflict tend to have greater adverse outcomes, longer hospitalizations (Schneiderman 2001), and a greater likelihood of medical–legal sequelae (Beckman et al. 1994; Halpern 2007). Thus, we would argue that our method, while somewhat more time intensive, is more cost-effective.

In Chap. 2, Integrating Theoretical Paradigms, we begin to provide the background for our approach to the difficult consultations, as we believe this foundational information is necessary to help the reader work best with his or her patients, their families, and other medical providers. We hope this chapter will augment the current methods of dealing with the difficult or complex patient and will provide insight that leads to better understanding of all the diverse aspects both of the people involved and their relationships. Moreover, in Chap. 2 we discuss how the

Fig. 1.1 Interrelated aspects
of the patient, the family and
the treatment team to be
considered in the
multidimensional approach to
a psychiatric consultation

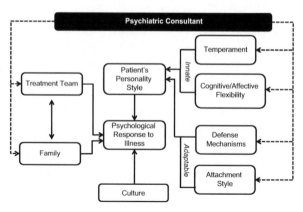

contemporary strategy will require the integration of what have historically been
viewed as conflicting approaches and theoretical orientations. For many, the tension
has been between the classic drive, conflict-based, object-relation, and one-person
psychology theories and the contemporary relational, intersubjective, co-
constructive, and two-person psychology theories. We believe this polarity is
unnecessary, as both psychodynamic theories have much to contribute to each
other and allow a person's place in the relational matrix to be rich and complex.
In Chap. 3, The Patient, we share an approach that is geared toward understanding
the patient *from the inside out* and describe a process of evaluating cognition,
cognitive flexibility, and temperament and then, with rich case examples, apply
these concepts to the complex patient in difficult consultations. In Chap. 4, we
approach The Family, portraying the way that family systems seek homeostasis,
even if, during the case of a serious medical or psychiatric illness, the homeostatic
equilibrium is achieved at the expense of alienating treatment-team members. In
this chapter, we introduce family systems concepts that may assist psychiatric
consultants with difficult or complex patients as well as with their families. Next,
in Chap. 5, The Treatment Team, we turn our attention to the medical providers
who care for these complex patients and explore the structure of the treatment team,
treatment-team conflicts, and core care concepts. This chapter also presents a
poignant vignette of "The noncompliant pediatric patient with a chronic medical
problem," which illustrates the in vivo application of these techniques. In Chap. 6,
Ethics, we review key ethical concepts and then, apply these principles to the
complex patient in difficult consultations. Chapter 7, The Culture, reviews psychological aspects of *culture shock*, a mourning process that is part of all difficult
consultations, whereby the patient learns to cope with the loss of the healthy self
and adjusts to the new role as patient. This chapter attends to different socioeconomic statuses that may interfere with providing care to the complex patient and
includes a section on the use of interpreters in the medical setting. It closes with a
review of the psychological issues related to immigration, language, and acculturation. Of course, we have not forgotten the newly minted clinician who may be asked
to present his or her patients or complex clinical cases at a Grand Rounds or in a

"case report" format, for which we have included Chap. 8, which comprises a helpful approach to these presentations of clinical material.

References

Beckman HB, Markakis KM, Suchman AL et al (1994) The doctor-patient relationship and malpractice. Lessons from plaintiff depositions. Arch Int Med 154(12):1365–1370

Bronheim HE, Fulop G, Kunkel EJ et al (1998) The academy of psychosomatic medicine practice guidelines for psychiatric consultation in the general medical setting. Psychosomatics 39(4): S8–S30

Dowling AS (2005) George Engel, MD (1913-1999). Am J Psychiatry 162:2039

Engel G (1977) The need for a new medical model: a challenge for biomedicine. Science 196 (4286):129–136

Engel GL (1980) The clinical application of the biopsychosocial model. Am J Psychiatry 137:535–544

Gabbard GO, Kay J (2001) The fate of integrated treatment: Whatever happened to the biopsychosocial psychiatrist? Am J Psychiatry 158(12):1956–1963

Gitlin DF, Levenson JL, Lyketsos CG (2004) Psychosomatic medicine: a new psychiatric subspecialty. Acad Psychiatry 28(1):4–11

Halpern J (2007) Empathy in patient-physician conflicts. J Gen Intern Med 22(5):696–700

Hamilton M (1959) The assessment of anxiety states by rating. Br J Med Psychol 32:50–55

Hamilton M (1960) A rating scale for depression. J Neurol Neurosurg Psychiatry 23:56–62

Hunter JJ, Maunder RG, Gupta M (2007) Teaching consultation-liaison psychotherapy: assessment of adaptation to medical and surgical illness. Acad Psychiatry 31:367–374

Kazak AE (2001) Comprehensive care for children with cancer and their families: a social ecological framework guiding research, practice, and policy. Child Ser Soc Pol Res Pract 4:217–233

Kontos N, Querques J, Freudenreich O (2006) The problem of the psychopharmacologist. Acad Psychiatry 30(3):218–226

Levenson JL (2002) Psychological factors affecting medical conditions. In: Hales RE, Yudovsky SC, Talbott JA (eds) The American psychiatric press textbook of psychiatry, 4th edn. American Psychiatric Press Incorporated, Washington, DC, pp 631–658

Lipowski ZJ (1983) Psychosocial reactions to physical illness. Can Med Assoc J 128:1069–1072

McIntyre JS (2002) A new subspecialty. Am J Psychiatry 159(12):1961–1963

Rush AJ, Gullion CM, Basco MR et al (1996) The inventory of depressive symptomatology (IDS): psychometric properties. Psychol Med 26:477–486

Schneiderman LJ (2001) Family demand for futile treatment. Med Ethics (Burlingt Mass) 3:8

Streltzer J, Hoyle L (2007) Interviewing in consultation-liaison psychiatry. Handbook of consultation-liaison psychiatry. Springer, New York, pp 387–393

Wei MH, Querques J, Stern TA (2011) Teaching trainees about the practice of consultation-liaison psychiatry in the general hospital. Psychiatry Clin North Am 34(3):689–707

Williams PD (1997) Siblings and pediatric chronic illness: a review of the literature. Int J Nurs Stud 34:312–323

Winnicott D (1964/1947) The child, the family, and the outside world. Penguin, Harmondsworth, England

Integrating Theoretical Paradigms

2

*The poor ego has a still harder time of it; it has to serve three
harsh masters, and it has to do its best to reconcile the claims
and demands of all three. . . . The three tyrants are the
external world, the superego, and the id*
—Sigmund Freud (1856–1939)

Having touched upon the history of the consultation process, we will now make a
brief sojourn to a number of psychological theories and the factors that influenced
their development. These theories will guide the consulting psychiatrist's approach
to the patient (Chap. 3), the family (Chap. 4), and the treatment team (Chap. 5).
Herein, we will provide the background for our approach to the complex psychiatric
case, which we hope will help the reader and psychiatric consultant gain insight into
the way human behaviors and relationships can be intertwined. Integrating what
have historically been viewed as conflicting approaches and theoretical
orientations, we aim to diffuse the tension that exists between the classic drive-
based, conflict-based, object-relations, and one-person psychology theories and the
contemporary relational, intersubjective, co-constructive, and two-person psychology theories, believing, as we do, that all of these have much to offer the psychiatric
consultant facing complex psychiatric cases. The consultant will likely be familiar
with terminology from classic and object-relations theories—learned during psychiatric training and/or routinely used in understanding patients and families—
however, the reader will also recognize in this chapter that the interventions
typically made in consultation-liaison work are more aligned with and guided by
contemporary, family-systems, and two-person psychological approaches defined
as a relational theory of mind, giving importance to both persons, co-constructing a
narrative influenced by the here and now (Aron 1990). The reader will also become
acquainted with the practical aspects of both classic and contemporary theories as
they apply to complex psychiatric patients and how they may be used in developing
interventions that promote stability and facilitate cooperation among the patient,
family, and treatment-team members.

S.V. Delgado and J.R. Strawn, *Difficult Psychiatric Consultations*,
DOI 10.1007/978-3-642-39552-9_2, © Springer-Verlag Berlin Heidelberg 2014

Certainly, any attempt to discuss psychodynamic theory in a book like this does a disservice to the many clinicians and theorists who have been instrumental in developing these theories. Nonetheless, for practical purposes, we will briefly review psychodynamic theories, and in doing so will highlight important concepts and processes that are particularly relevant to difficult consultations. Importantly, we will not address the controversies surrounding the process of psychodynamic formulations using classic, one-person psychology and contemporary relational, two-person psychologies. Instead, we refer the reader to contemporary sources that present these controversies in a balanced manner (BPCG 2010; Fonagy et al. 2002; Greenberg 2003; Mitchell 2003; Wachtel 2011).

Before we begin our discussion proper of psychodynamic theory and its genesis, we should note that we have organized this chapter around what is often referred to as "one-person" and "two-person" psychologies. The astute reader will already be aware that these terms fail to capture the complexities of each psychotherapeutic approach. At the most basic level, one-person psychology tends to focus on the patient's understanding, within the therapeutic encounter, of his or her past experiences as they relate to intrapsychic processes transferred onto the therapist. By contrast, two-person psychology may be seen as focusing symmetrically on both players (i.e., the therapist and the patient), and the treatment is considered to occur through a relational here-and-now constructivism rather than through intrapsychic shifts based on the patient's experience as perceived by a neutral therapist. In many cases, the therapist employing a two-person psychology may be less reticent, less neutral, more likely to use implicit and explicit disclosure, and may welcome enactments in the treatment of his or her patients.

2.1   Classic Psychonanlytic Theories: One-Person Psychology

Drive Theory

Classic psychoanalytic theory was developed by Sigmund Freud (1856–1939), who based his theories on his psychoanalytic work with adult patients. In his efforts to understand the human mind, Freud proposed several hypotheses. First, the *topographic model* (Fig. 2.1) posits that most mental life occurs in the *unconscious,* and that *preconscious and conscious* life is rather limited. Later, in revising the *topographic model*, Freud developed the *structural model* (Fig. 2.2). In this model the unconscious is comprised of several intrapsychic agencies: (1) the id, which embodies the instinctual sexual and aggressive drives; (2) the superego, which consists of the cultural and societal norms that have been incorporated into the person's psyche; and (3) the ego, which moderates conflict between the id (which desires free reign) and the superego (which urges civility). Still later Freud wrote about the importance of the sexual drive theory in the form of psychosexual developmental phases determined by the organ of predominant interest to the

Fig. 2.1 Sigmund Freud's
topographic model of the
mind

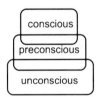

Fig. 2.2 Sigmund Freud's
topographic and structural
model of the mind

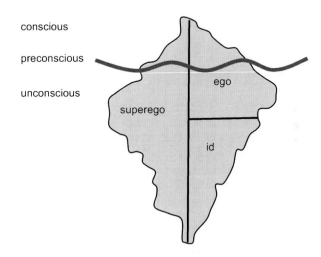

Table 2.1 Sigmund Freud's model of psychosexual development

Psychosexual stage	Oral		Anal	Oedipal	Genital	Latency	
Age	0–6 months	18 months	24 months	4 years	4–6 years	7–11 years	Adolescence

infant/child for pleasure. Freud posited that the key developmental task of children involved "taming the instinctual drives" of the id through the development of the superego and ego (Freud 1916–1917). As can be seen in Table 2.1, there are three phases (oral, anal, and phallic) of the developmental process—often referred to as *psychosexual development*—and each requires that conflicts from the previous phase be successfully resolved. Freud emphasized that during the phallic phase, between the ages of 4 through 6 years, the intrapsychic conflict centers on the important oedipal complex, part of a longitudinal process of psychosexual development. When the anxieties of the oedipal complex are resolved, the person achieves the healthy psychological genital phase of normal heterosexuality (Freud 1924). According to Freud, pleasurable heterosexual intercourse was the goal of his psychosexual theories: "the subordination of all the component sexual instincts under the primacy of the genitals" (Freud 1905).

For Freud, unresolved conflicts of the oral, anal, or oedipal phase lead the person to have a neurotic fixation that, when he or she is under stress, manifests in a regression of ego functions to behaviors of the phase fixated in. Additionally, classic Freudian theory posits that a given personality is determined (or defined) by the ego functions that he or she utilizes and is continually influenced by the superego, which inhibits the unconscious drives' press for gratification.

A summary of Freud's theories and their importance to psychoanalysis can be found in *An Elementary Textbook of Psychoanalysis* by Charles Brenner (1974) and in the more recent work, *Freud and Beyond*, by Mitchell and Black (1995).

Ego Psychology

Heinz Hartman (1894–1970), a psychiatrist and psychoanalyst, often described as one of Freud's favorite students, developed the school of ego psychology. Holding that the ego has a biological substrate that includes perception, memory, concentration, motor coordination, and learning, he believed these innate ego capacities had autonomy from the sexual and aggressive drives of the id and were not products of frustration or conflict. Hartman coined the term "autonomous ego functions" (Hartman 1958), and his ideas share much with recent concepts concerning implicit memory systems and internal working schema stored in non-declarative memory systems (Mancia 2006).

The window into a personality style can be created through the study and understanding of the ego defense mechanisms an individual employs in coping with daily-life anxiety and threats to self-esteem from intrapsychic conflicts. Though Sigmund Freud was the first to describe such defense mechanisms, our contemporary understanding of these processes comes from his daughter, Anna Freud (1895–1982), who systematically classified these defenses, compiling a comprehensive catalog in her classic work *The Ego and the Mechanisms of Defense* (Freud 1937/1966). Sometimes we might consciously know which defense mechanisms we use in relation to others—as in humor to manage family conflict or denying or overlooking a colleague's negative comments—but in most cases they occur unconsciously. Defense mechanisms usually are adaptive and can have a salutary effect, allowing an individual to function normally. Importantly, however, when used in a repetitive fashion, defense mechanisms can become maladaptive and induce further anxiety. In this regard, a diabetic patient who unconsciously and routinely uses denial may avoid following through with the treatment team's recommendations regarding monitoring blood sugar and administering insulin, and thus his or her diabetes may be poorly controlled. This distinction between adaptive and maladaptive defense mechanisms was thoroughly evaluated by George Vaillant, MD (1934–) in his seminal work *Ego Mechanisms of Defense: A Guide for Clinicians and Researchers* (Vaillant 1992), in which he hierarchically categorizes defense mechanisms as mature, neurotic, immature, and pathological

Table 2.2 Common defense mechanisms

Category	Defense mechanism	Description
Immature and pathological	Acting out	Unhealthy behavioral responses to an intolerable wish that bring partial relief
	Denial	Reality is not accepted as it is too painful
	Projection	Attributing unacceptable thoughts or feelings to someone or something else
	Projective identification	An individual's projections exert interpersonal pressure which induces the other person to unconsciously identify with what has been projected
	Splitting	Others are experienced as "all good" or "all bad" and ambivalence is not tolerated.
Neurotic	Regression	Reverting to an earlier, less mature way of managing conflicted feelings and stress
	Repression	Burying a painful feeling or thought from awareness, though it may resurface in symbolic form
	Isolation of affect	Detaching the affect from an unpleasant thought or behavior
	Displacement	Channeling a feeling or thought from its actual source to something or someone that is more acceptable
	Reaction formation	Adopting beliefs, attitudes, and feelings that are contrary to an unacceptable wish
	Rationalization	Justifying unacceptable behaviors and motivations by "good" and acceptable rational explanations
Mature	Altruism	Placing the needs of others before the needs of oneself
	Humor	An unpleasant thought or experience is viewed as comedic to buffer the unpleasant affect
	Sublimation	Redirecting unacceptable, instinctual drives into healthy and socially acceptable channels
	Suppression	The act of consciously setting aside and controlling unacceptable thoughts or feelings

(Table 2.2). More recently, these defense mechanisms have been categorized dichotomously into mature and immature based on the degree to which they are considered pathologic.

Having briefly discussed Freud's psychoanalytic models and related ego-psychological models, which will be of practical relevance to the psychiatrist working with difficult consultations, we will now discuss three important concepts: *introjection, transference, countertransference*. These concepts subtend classical psychodynamic and contemporary psychodynamic theories and are central to approaching the consultation with complex psychiatric patients.

Introjection

Vignette: Healthy Introjection
A sibling with parental healthy introjections reassures her hospitalized brother, who is receiving treatment for newly diagnosed diabetes, stating, "Everything will be ok. I will help you feel better."

Vignette: Unhealthy Introjection
An adolescent patient with cystic fibrosis refuses to complete respiratory treatments and accuses the treatment-team members of being "mean and stupid like my parents." Her reaction is based on unhealthy introjected parents, confirmed as the parents do not provide emotional support during the adolescent's hospital stay and yell that, if she does not improve, it is her fault.

Introjection refers to the internalization of psychological characteristics that a child attributes to caregiving, parental figures, yet that are filtered by the child's internal wishes and needs (Delgado and Songer 2009). As an example, introjection of positive early childhood experiences is evinced when psychologically healthy children and adults who experience an acute medical problem (see vignette) allow for an also healthy loved one to reassure them, providing in an empathic manner their support to continue with the medical course recommended by the treatment team. On the flip side, when the patient has been a victim of neglect or abuse, they may unconsciously be loyal to the introjection of bad-object (negative experience) representations and, unable to psychologically access a healthier internal experience to interpret the situations, are likely to recreate/repeat early experiences in which they were criticized for "being bad." In the clinical setting, this individual is inclined to believe that members of a treatment team dislike him or her, particularly when the team attempts to set limits on the use of medications for pain or the number of visitors allowed. Further, these patients frequently see the treatment team as inflicting pain, which sets the stage for a pattern of refusing treatment recommendations and of misinterpreting good intentions.

Transference

Vignette: Transference
A patient with history of being passive and dependent, who was raised by critical and demanding parents whom he feared, is unable to make crucial decisions to continue with the treatment recommendations. The patient feels pressured by the requests of the treatment-team members for decisions by him or her, and the perception of their authority leads to passivity and indecision in spite of efforts to reassure the patient of the likely good outcome from the treatment.

For much of the twentieth century, Sigmund Freud's process of transference, considered central to psychoanalysis and psychodynamic psychotherapy, was felt to be a critical element for psychotherapeutic change to occur. In short, the phenomenon involves the transferring of early, unresolved wishes and feelings toward parents or caregivers onto the therapist or another who has attributes that remind the patient of these early unconscious experiences. By remembering and repeating with the therapist these unhealthy patterns, the patient's conflicts are "worked through" in the psychotherapeutic process (Freud 1914). Upon experiencing improvement in the symptoms that brought him or her to treatment, the patient starts making more mature life choices. Through the "interpretation" of transference, the individual's previously unconscious conflicts and maladaptive experiences are brought to consciousness, resulting in the patient developing insight and improving symptomatically. Currently, an understanding of transference is helpful for the psychiatric consultant in assessing the back-and-forth interactions between patients and treatment-team members during difficult psychiatric consultations.

Countertransference

Vignette: Countertransference
A 40-year-old man hospitalized with asthma responds in an angry manner to his physician at the need to take maintenance medication for his condition. The physician has a history of difficulties with conflict when working with patients, as these current experiences resonate with past discord with siblings. The physician begins to round in the early morning, when the patient has just awoken, to limit interaction and avoid conflict. Thus his countertransference is being acted out.

Countertransference occurs when the therapist unwittingly participates in the patient's transference. His or her unconscious reactions to the patient guide the therapist's responses, which are rooted in the therapist's own unresolved intrapsychic conflicts evoked by the patient. The issue of countertransference has direct relevance to the psychiatric consultant and has been well described in the extant literature. In his classic paper "Taking care of the hateful patient," Groves notes, "admitted or not, the fact remains that a few patients kindle aversion, fear, despair or even downright malice in their doctors" (Groves 1978). Groves believes that the negative feelings some physicians have for hateful patients are the result of countertransference. If the physician's actions are influenced by these negative reactions, a countertransference enactment ensues by which the physician gratifies the transference wishes of the patient. In such cases, the clinician may find that recognizing his or her countertransference reactions will help to avoid many clinical pitfalls, as discussed in Chap. 5.

Object Relations Theory

From the 1940s to the 1960s, psychoanalytic theorists increasingly recognized the importance of the patient's early interactions with parents and caregivers, given that these developmental experiences were crucial to the formation of the individual's ego. As a result, in the 1940s a natural transition from *ego psychology* to *object-relations theory* evolved. Melanie Klein (1882–1960), a student of Freud, is thought to be the first object-relations theorist, noting that object relations were at the center of a person's emotional life (Klein 1932). Object relations refers to the capacity to have a stable and rewarding relationships based on the internalization (a process closely related to introjection as described above) of the early childhood representations of others in the form of "objects." However, internalization of these objects is not a mere imitation. Filtered by the child's wishes and needs (Delgado and Songer 2009), these objects are attributed an individualized significance. The variability in what an infant innately happens to internalize from his or her parents as "objects" supported later psychodynamic theories that incorporated temperament and attachment styles into what has recently been termed "intersubjectivity." Clinically, this concept—intersubjectivity—has been defined as "the capacity to share, know, understand, empathize with, feel, participate in, resonate with, enter into the lived subjective experience of another" and "interpreting overt behaviors such as posture, tone of voice, speech rhythm and facial expression, as well as verbal content . . . which assumes that [the therapist] can come to share, know, and feel what is in the mind of the patient and the sense of what the patient is experiencing" (Stern 2004).

   Melanie Klein posits that the infant, as part of a normative developmental phase, from 0 to 4 months of age, possesses a primitive fear. During this period, which Klein refers to as the *paranoid position,* internalized representations of caregivers are experienced as part objects that are split into "good" and "bad" objects (e.g., the loving mother, nurturing mother, and the depriving mother). In the early stages, the child maintains the self and object split to avoid the distress in recognizing that there are aggressive and depriving aspects of the self as well as the other. Then, from 4 to 12 months of age, the child learns to integrate and tolerate that a person has both "good" and "bad" parts and enters a healthy phase that Klein describes as *the depressive position* (Klein 1932). Having psychologically achieved the depressive position, the child proceeds to develop a capacity of concern for others and guilt about one's actions and thoughts about others, with desire for reparation (Winnicott 1965). Klein believed that individuals who are unable to work through the depressive position in their childhood continue to struggle to relate to others in adult life. More recently, the contemporary object relations theorist and psychoanalyst Otto Kernberg, MD (1928–), has suggested that when the patient's internal representation of others remains "split," they primarily use low-level defense mechanisms including splitting, projection, and projective identification (Kernberg 1976). According to Kernberg, these patients were best understood as exhibiting a borderline level of organization, with poor capacity for affect regulation, and are prone to impulsive actions, including suicide (Kernberg 2000). Those with borderline-level organization have tumultuous relationships with others, unconsciously experiencing them as "bad objects" that evoke early internalized frightening and chaotic experiences, usually at the hands of a critical parent or caregiver. They often display maladaptive defense mechanisms—splitting, projection and projective identification, and these are commonly linked to patients with longstanding patterns of difficult/feisty temperaments, poor cognitive and affective flexibility (see Chap. 3), and insecure attachment styles (described below). In turn, these patients are unable to navigate the back-and-forth complex adjustments to different affective states of the other. Further, they have a limited capacity to have genuine concern for others and little or no guilt about their thoughts and interactions with them.

It would be beyond the scope of this book to provide a full description of all the object-relation processes of individuals with character pathology. We focus instead on the theory's most relevant clinical contributions in working with difficult psychiatric consultations. To this end, we define splitting, projection and projective identification.

Projection

Projection refers to the ego defense mechanism whereby an individual reduces the anxiety in recognizing some of his or her own negative attributes, desires, and emotions by unconsciously ascribing them onto another person (Akhtar 2009). At first glance, the process may seem much like Freud's transference. However, projection occurs when a person projects his or her own state of mind onto a new object (e.g., therapist or treatment-team member), whereas in transference the past parental experiences are being repeated with the therapist or treatment-team member standing in for the parental object.

Projective Identification

Projective identification involves two components: (1) projection as described above, in which the person blames the other by projecting onto him or her the individual's own unconscious object representations of the self, which they cannot tolerate as being their own, and (2) the negative reactions by the "recipient" of the person's projections which "exerts interpersonal pressure that nudges the other person to...[unconsciously identify with that which has been projected]" (Gabbard 2010). Importantly, though the recipient's behaviors are generally not considered "in character" but rather are a reaction to the feelings that belong to the person projecting, these very reactions, inability to contain and tolerate the affective states evoked by the projections, he or she will identify with the projections and uncharacteristic negative behaviors ensue. Sadly they confirm what the patient believed to be the case all along. An example in a clinical setting: a physician who is well-liked has a pleasant temperament and is generally able to connect with others, attends a family meeting, and is accused by the patient's family of not treating the patient or family fairly and of dismissing their feelings. Initially, the physician recognizes this is not the case and, with compassion, attempts to explain to the patient and family that they are being treated fairly and that their feelings are important to him and to his treatment team. Yet the physician's explanation infuriates the patient and his family, who feel that their experience is being further rejected. They continue with the projections, and at some point, without being consciously aware; the treating physician incorporates the projected attributes and begins to react in an uncharacteristic way. He becomes overly firm, insisting on strict boundaries and defending himself and his treatment team. In short, the physician has now manifested what the patient and family accused him of; he is dismissive and treats them in a harsh manner. It is common for a person caught up in identifying with a patient's projections to end meetings abruptly and later ask the team, "What just happened?" Typically team members say, "The patient got under your skin. It's not like you."

As with many psychodynamic or psychoanalytic theoretical concepts, projective identification and countertransference remain subjects of controversy. Certainly, both represent the reactions of the healthcare provider when he or she is the recipient of a displaced conflict or projections from a patient, and they may share other psychological facets as well. As American psychiatrist and psychoanalyst Glen Gabbard (1949–) notes, "the similarities between projective identification as used in contemporary psychoanalytic writing, role-responsiveness, and countertransference enactment have been observed by a number of authors" (Gabbard and Wilkinson 1994). For many, the difference between the two related concepts derives from the theoretical school that spawned them. The classic drive-theory school positions countertransference in relation to the unconscious conflicts with early objects, conflicts that are repeated when the patient transfers/displaces past experiences onto the recipient. In the school of object relations, projective identification is a primitive phenomenon in which the patient psychologically forces the disavowed bad self-object onto a recipient who unconsciously returns the foreign bad self-object back to the patient as if the recipient had owned it. Some contemporary authors believe these two mechanisms are, for practical purposes, one and the same (Renik 2004).

Splitting

The phenomenon commonly referred to as "splitting" is categorized, in the hierarchy of defense mechanisms, as pathological. There are some difficulties in defining and understanding splitting when the origin of this concept is studied. There is splitting of the ego, which Freud described in his early work (Freud 1938), although the predominant view is Klein's splitting of the self as a part of the developmental stage in infants. Splitting, therefore, is a metapsychological concept with many interpretations in object-relations theory. Put simply, we define splitting as the inability to hold in mind that the person in a relationship is a whole entity with both positive and negative attributes. When it becomes unconsciously intolerable for a patient to accept that the person he or she experiences as depriving or abusive also has positive characteristics, splitting occurs. In order to modulate his or her inability to integrate and view himself and others as a whole objects with strengths and weakness, the patient resorts to the use of primitive ego defense mechanisms and, like the infant, "splits their self and other object representation into good and bad, self and other objects" (Delgado and Songer 2009). This process prevents any form of closeness, as the relationship is now distorted and no longer bound by reality.

An example of splitting is when a patient experiences a physician as being the best they have ever met and several days later, following a perceived transgression (being late to bedside rounds, encountering a treatment complication, etc.), sees the same physician as inattentive to his or her needs. In such cases, the patient is unable to reconcile the situation and thus unable to forgive the physician for his transgression (Horwitz 2005). The patient experiences the physician as becoming identical to his or her unconsciously held bad object and, as such, the patient may escalate his or her negative behavior, impeding psychological proximity for fear of retaliation. Unfortunately, the term splitting in the colloquial sense is commonly misused by psychiatrists, physicians, and other healthcare providers to describe situations in which patients are pleasant with one physician and angry or belligerent toward another. Although this occurs often in hospital settings, which we will discuss throughout this book, this is actually a process of projection, as described earlier, rather than splitting.

Let us clarify this distinction by way of everyday examples. We often see sports fans boasting that their team is the best (in other words, the team is "all good"), and this sense may be accentuated if the fan has a particular personal connection to the team (e.g., if they have a child or friend playing on it). In this example, the opposing team is disliked and thought of as "bad." We see here all of the elements of *projection*: idealized positive aspects of the self are projected onto the home-team players, and negative aspects of the self are projected onto the opposing team. We now use a similar example to illustrate *splitting*. Say during the sports event, a fan notices his or her team-making mistakes. The fan experiences the mistakes as personal and begins to distort the situation, believing the coaches should be listening to what he or she has been yelling regarding plays. He feels frustrated when the plays he's calling are not adopted and is suddenly unable to view the matter realistically. Moreover, the fan may be unable to see that the opposing team, at that time, is actually playing better. Thus, the home team is now viewed as a depriving the fan, in not giving the fan the win he deserves, and is therefore not worthy of the fan's support. In this instance, it is necessary for the fan, who is splitting, to have history of employing primitive defense mechanisms with projections of the depriving early parental objects, without being able to experience healthy ambivalence about others. This type of fan—as we often see in the news media—is prone to acting out against the players and coaches, may yell obscenities, throw objects, and unfortunately at times resort to violence. In contrast, the "healthy" fan who is upset if their team plays poorly does not experience the loss as personal and merely hopes for a better game next time. This healthy fan has the capacity to hold in mind that teams normally have good and bad games, and he or she is able to integrate the team as a "whole object."

A similar everyday example, likely more familiar to those who have treated patients with psychodynamic psychotherapy, is when a person develops a crush on a friend at a social event. First, the person excitedly admires the positive attributes of the friend—polite, funny, and serious about succeeding in their career. When the feelings of excitement influence their perception of the friend, the person begins to project internal good-object representations. The projections are made with the idyllic hope/belief that the friend will have attributes similar to their own—love the same type of music, social causes, food, etc.—thus, the belief is that the friend seems to have the makings of a soul mate. This is typical of the early phase of romantic friendships, which are influenced by both the real attributes of the people involved as well as the hoped-for attributes, which are projected. Weeks later, the person, who also loves pets, finds that the possible soul mate actually strongly dislikes all pets. If the person is psychologically healthy and not prone to splitting, he or she will recognize that, as a whole, their friend is not perfect and the positive qualities of altruism and humor outweigh their flaw in the lack of interest for pets, which will be negotiated over time. When the person is prone to such primitive defense mechanisms as splitting, the discovery that the friend dislikes pets results in sudden anger, and he or she may state, "I knew it couldn't be true, and you are a stupid jerk. If you don't like pets, you don't know anything about love." They feel personally rejected and proceed to end the relationship. They have been unable to hold in mind their friend as a "whole object" with good and bad characteristics.

While we have attempted to introduce the reader to the nuances of splitting and projection, we recognize that, at times, splitting is a very complex intrapsychic process. While a full discussion of its subtleties is beyond the scope of this book, we refer the reader to several important and detailed descriptions of this concept by many object-relations theorists (i.e., Otto Kernberg 2000; James Masterson 2005; Donald Rinsley 1982).

Self Psychology

Like Freud, the American psychoanalyst Heinz Kohut (1913–1981) based his theory of self-psychology on inferences made during the treatment of adult patients. He hypothesized that narcissistic disorders of the self were due to childhood parental empathic failures (Kohut 1971). Kohut proposed that there were healthy and unhealthy forms of narcissism, in contrast to Freud, who considered narcissism a pathological investment of the ego by the sexual drive (Freud 1920). Kohut believed that treating disorders of the self, required a therapeutic empathic

Fig. 2.3 Common personality types of difficult patients according to Groves (1978)

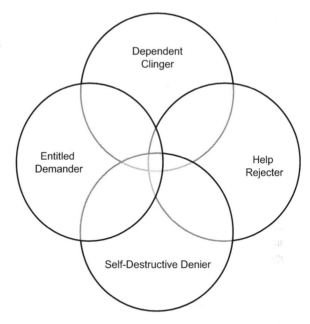

reparation by the analyst of the patient's maladaptive (idealizing, mirroring, and twinship "self-object") functions. "Empathic failure" is the term used to describe a situation in which a patient feels misunderstood by the therapist, as is seen in the case of Jason in Chap. 3 (McLean 2007).

Personality Types

In two controversial papers, Groves (1978) and Strous et al. (2006) posit that the "difficult" and/or "hateful patients" encountered in medical centers may be categorized into four personality subtypes: (1) dependent clingers, (2) entitled demanders, (3) manipulative help-rejecters, and (4) self-destructive deniers (Fig. 2.3). They further suggest interventions for the physician in helping the patients in each of the four categories, to mitigate negative countertransference reactions. Strous et al. conclude "understanding of this "hateful" patient will lead to improved physician well-being and satisfaction, less self-destructive patient behavior, improved treatment compliance, and a lower risk of litigation." These personality types derive from observable traits to the general physician and do not represent the classification of personality disorders described in the *Diagnostic and Statistical Manual of Mental Disorders* 5th Edition (American Psychiatric Association 2013), where the traits must be part of enduring patterns that emerge under a wide range of situations and not only in the hospital setting. Using the concept of personality types may help the consulting psychiatrist to discuss with the treatment team patterns of behavior and thinking of patients who fit one of the above categories.

Personality Disorders

The psychiatric consultant is best prepared when understanding personality disorders and personality patterns mitigating the negative effects in difficult psychiatric consultations. It has been estimated that 20 % of patients seen by a psychiatric consultant have a personality disorder (Laugharne 2013). A patient with a personality disorder typically has difficulties providing a reliable and accurate timeline in terms of the symptom presentation.

In the *Diagnostic and Statistical Manual of Mental Disorders 4th Edition, Text-Revision* (*DSM-IV-TR*, American Psychiatric Association 2000), personality disorders were included in Axis II of the multiaxial diagnostic approach. Additionally, personality disorders are described as having "an enduring pattern of inner experience and behavior that deviates markedly from the expectations of the individual's culture, is pervasive and inflexible, has an onset in adolescence or early adulthood, is stable over time, and leads to distress or impairment" (American Psychiatric Association 2000). In the *DSM-IV-TR*, ten personality disorders are outlined and categorized in three clusters: A, B, and C. In consultation psychiatry, we have found that patients with three personality disorders from cluster B (borderline personality disorder, histrionic personality disorder, and narcissistic personality disorder) are the most difficult for treatment teams to understand and to engage effectively. Despite the challenges of working with those who exhibit a personality disorder, however, it is important to recognize that these patients may also have brief periods of lucidity and tempered social engagement, seen when they interact with certain persons (e.g., individuals in distress, those who are experiencing vulnerability). A patient with a predominant personality disorder may also evince characteristics of the other personality disorders types (Fig. 2.4) or may have an amalgam of several types of each personality. We should note that in the *Diagnostic and Statistical Manual of Mental Disorders 5th Edition* (*DSM-5* 2013) personality disorders are captured in the same categorical model and criteria for the ten personality disorders included in *DSM-IV-TR*, although there was a removal of the multiaxial system and the documentation of diagnosis is in a non-axial format, combining the former Axes I, II, and III with what have often been considered primary disorders (e.g., major depressive disorder, generalized anxiety disorder, etc.). Though it is too early to know what the implications of this change are on the level of diagnosis and treatment, the psychiatric consultant is nevertheless best prepared when understanding the personality disorders and patterns that can be helpful in mitigating negative effects during consultations.

Fig. 2.4 Overlap between "normal" and "disordered" personality patterns. Importantly, there are shared features, common internal experiences, and common patterns of relating among the "classic" personality disorders, wherein even the "borderline" patient may occasionally struggle with "narcissistic" or "histrionic" difficulties and may also—at times—relate in a more "normal" manner

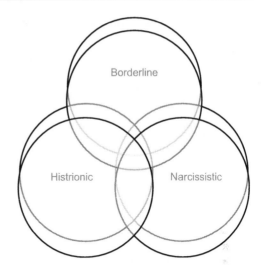

Mentalization

Vignette: Mentalization

A 2 1/2 year old girl is playing a simple board game and attempts to win by jumping several spaces ahead. She sheepishly looks at her mother to see if this has been noticed. Her mother returns a "hmmm" disapproving look. The child infers her mother's intent, desire and feelings and begins to laugh as she retraces the path of her game character on the board and says "Oh dear," indicating her awareness that this was "not right."

Contemporary theorists believe that the central problem of patients with personality disorders is their difficulty with the ability to mentalize (Allen et al. 2008). This process involves the ability to interpret behavior as meaningful and as based on the mental states and psychological makeup of both the self and others, such as desires, needs, beliefs, reasons, and feelings. Some have said this is akin to "holding mind in mind" (Allen et al. 2008). It is accepted that persons with a history of being securely attached have good mentalizing abilities, while a person who grew insecurely attached has difficulty mentalizing and makes use of maladaptive defense mechanisms. Mentalization-based treatment (MBT) is becoming widely recognized as helpful for patients with personality disorders in both adolescents (Rossouw and Fonagy 2012) and adults (Bateman and Fonagy 2008, 2009). Yet the idea of a mentalization-focused treatment is "the least novel therapeutic approach imaginable, simply because it revolves around a fundamental human capacity—indeed, the capacity that makes us human" (Allen and Fonagy 2006).

2.2   Relational Theories: Two-Person Psychology

Although the work by two-person theorists or "relationalists" has been frowned upon by some, it has served to provide clarity about the application of attachment-theory tenets in psychotherapy and psychoanalysis. We find that these principles are very useful for our day-to-day clinical work in the hospital setting, especially in navigating impasses in complex psychiatric cases. Below we will provide brief reviews of the relevant concepts from each theory followed by examples in which they are utilized in difficult psychiatric consultations. We will again cherry pick the main concepts of contemporary theories to give the reader a basic understanding of their importance and applicability.

Attachment Theory

John Bowlby (1907–1990), a British psychiatrist and psychoanalyst, is best known for his contributions to our understanding of the process of attachment. As such, he is considered the "father of attachment theory"—though Bowlby may have preferred to be known as the "the primary caregiver of attachment theory," which would reflect his belief that an infant needs to develop a relationship with at least one primary caregiver, regardless of gender, for healthy psychological development to occur. Bowlby departed from traditional psychoanalytic school of thought when he discovered through his work that infants have an evolutionary, innate wish for close, shared experiences with their primary caregivers for survival, growth, and development (Bowlby 1999). He felt this urge was biologically rooted and divorced from Freud's drive theory, which placed emphasis on sexuality and aggression as innate drives (Freud 1916-1917). Bowlby notes that early in life, the infant creates attachment behavioral systems that help it assess whether its caregiver is available not only physically but emotionally. He further suggests that the quality of the attachment between the infant and the parent or primary caregiver is a powerful predictor of a child's later social and emotional facility (Benoit 2004). The caregiver strongly influences how the infant develops the capacity for emotional regulation of their feelings, creating an "internal working model of social relationships" that serves as a template when relating to others (Bowlby 1999). Attachment theory subsequently provided a longitudinal view on how early dyadic relationships, with mother or primary caregivers, shape the quality of emotional relationships the child has with others throughout its lifespan.

During the 1960s and 1970s, developmental psychologist Mary Ainsworth (1913–1999), influenced by her communication with John Bowlby, began to experimentally evaluate his basic formulations through studies of infant–parent pairs in Scotland and Uganda (Ainsworth et al. 1978). Her work led to the foundation of different descriptions of patterns of attachment between infants and caregivers based on observable traits of the mother and the infant during times of separation and reunification: (1) secure attachment, (2) avoidant attachment, and (3) anxious attachment (Ainsworth et al. 1978). Ainsworth's work was later expanded by Mary Main (1943–), a researcher who introduced the concept of "disorganized attachment," which was instrumental in understanding the experiences of children exposed to chaotic and unpredictable environments had and their tendency to seek the same type of interactions (Main 2000).

Attachment Styles

The four attachment styles described above warrant further discussion, given the central role they play in determining the patient's ability to interact with the treatment team and with regard to the ways they can be used to guide the interventions the psychiatric consultant may chose, as discussed later in this book (Table 2.3).

Secure Attachment
The first type of attachment, secure attachment, occurs when the infant is cared for by a person who provides a sense of safety and reciprocity. The caregiver also exhibits empathic attunement and helps the infant handle normal periods of distress with actions such as holding, soothing with touch, rocking rhythmically, or singing with a melodic voice. The child develops with a coherent discourse over time, values attachments whether pleasant or temporarily unpleasant, and is able to provide others a sense of reciprocity.

Ambivalent Attachment (Anxious)
The ambivalent type of attachment occurs when the infant feels anxious because the caregiver's availability is unpredictable and inconsistent. The infant develops patterns of relationships based on superficiality. The ambivalent infant grows to be a child and adult that wishes for closeness with others, but often fails to convey a sense of reciprocity and as a result is frequently rejected, repeating the original pattern established with caregiver.

Avoidant Attachment (Dismissive)
The avoidant type of attachment occurs when the infant is in constant fear due to the unpredictability of the quality of the relationship with the caregiver and cannot develop a stable internal working model of social relationships (Bowlby 1999). As the infant grows, he or she shows a tendency toward passivity and avoids the expression of affect with others to prevent feelings of rejection and to protect against the hurt of being ignored. The avoidant infant as a child and adult develops patterns of self-sufficiency and independence and consequently has difficulties with closeness.

Disorganized Attachment
Disorganized attachment occurs when the infant experiences caregivers lack of coherent attachment patterns and relate with a poor sense of reciprocity. There is common history of abandonment or trauma in these children, who grow to be frightened of commitment and have significant vulnerabilities that prevent them from sustaining stable relationships, causing a repeating cycle of their incoherent life discourse. As adults they are prone to trauma and dissociative experiences. Some believe this an early precursor of borderline personality disorders.

Table 2.3 Attachment patterns in children and their caregivers' responses

Attachment pattern	Child's behaviors	Caregiver behaviors
Secure	• Uses caregiver as a secure base for exploration. • Protests caregiver's departure and seeks proximity and is comforted on return, returning to exploration. • May be comforted by a stranger, although shows clear preference for the caregiver.	• Responds appropriately, promptly and consistently to child's needs. • Caregiver has successfully formed a secure parental attachment bond to the child.
Ambivalent(anxious)	• Unable to use caregiver as a secure base. • Distressed on separation with ambivalence, anger, and on return of caregiver, has reluctance to warm and return to play. • Preoccupied with caregiver's availability, seeking contact but resisting angrily when it is achieved. • Not easily calmed by stranger. In this relationship, the child feels anxious as the caregiver's availability has not been consistent.	• Inconsistent between appropriate and anxious responses. • Generally will only respond after increased attachment behavior from the infant. • Caregiver is reluctant to warm and return to play with child.
Avoidant (dismissive)	• During play there is little affective sharing. • Little or no distress on departure, little or no visible response to return, ignoring or turning away with no effort to maintain contact if picked up. • Treats the stranger similarly to the caregiver. • The child behaves in a rebellious manner and grows to have a lower self-image and self-esteem.	• During play there is little affective sharing • Little or no response to distressed child. • Discourages crying and encourages independence.
Disorganized	• Stereotypies on return such as freezing or rocking. • Lack of coherent attachment strategy shown by contradictory, disoriented behaviors such as approaching but with the back turned.	• Frightened or frightening behavior, intrusiveness, withdrawal, negativity, role confusion, affective communication errors and at times maltreatment.

Summary regarding patterns infants have in strange situation and corresponding patterns of Adult Attachment classification
Descriptions are adapted from Main et al. (1985), Main and Goldwyn (1984, 1998), Ainsworth et al. (1978) and Main and Solomon (1990)

Attachment Theory Across Lifespan

Attachment theory has contributed to the understanding of how early childhood experiences contribute to, not just child attachment patterns, but to attachment patterns of adults across their life spans. Shaver and Hazan (1988) eloquently describe the connection between early attachment patterns and characteristics of later romantic relationships. These studies suggest that adults who describe themselves as having secure, avoidant, or ambivalent styles of attachment in their current relationships had similar patterns as children in their families of origin. Moreover, attachment research has recently has broadened its focus; these approaches are now being used to inform novel psychotherapeutic treatments and to enhance our understanding of interpersonal dynamics in marital relationships, among middle-aged adults and among the elderly (Cicirelli 1991, 1998; Weiss 1982, 1991).

For Parkes et al. (1991), the scope is broader yet. According to him, a healthy society depends on factors that (1) minimize disruptive events, (2) protect each child's attachment experience with caregivers from harm, and (3) support families in coping with obstacles in their lives. In addition, Parkes emphasizes the importance of social context on the growth of the infant and suggests that safeguarding the infant's dyadic relationships can have further implications in public health: "valuing of attachment relations thus has public policy and moral implications for society, not just psychological implications for attachment dyads" (Bretherton 1992).

Attachment Theory in the Medical Setting

Having described how the bidirectional attachment process involving the infant or child and the caregiver sets the stage for "lifelong patterns of stress-response, receptivity to social support and vulnerability to illness" (Maunder and Hunter 2001), we turn our attention to its role in the difficult psychiatric consultation. Patients in the medical setting with a history of secure attachment will have a sense of safety about the services provided by their treatment team (Sullivan et al. 2009), whereas those with insecure attachment styles will exhibit mistrust toward the treatment team and may be hesitant to follow its recommendations. Encountering this mistrust, team members may in turn engage in negative interactions with the patient based on their counter-transference reactions (Miller and Katz 1989). Understanding attachment theory can help the psychiatric consultant in this setting address the behaviors of all parties involved. And by providing the treatment-team members with a useful framework for assessment—giving them the understanding that the quality of the patient's early attachment has established patterns that will be repeated in their encounters with medical providers—the clinician and the team can more ably effect the patient's adherence to treatment (Hooper et al. 2011). Hooper et al further add that "Attachment theory may provide a blueprint for attachment-based practice in the context of medical settings. This blueprint or guide can help physicians better understand and respond to the ways in which patients' presenting symptomatology are described and discussed, and the manner in which patients form relationships and interact with other significant persons, including healthcare providers (e.g., primary care physicians, nurses, psychologists, psychiatrists)" (2011).

2.3   Social Referencing, Affective Attunement, and Intersubjectivity

In recent years, neurodevelopmentally informed research has extended the works by Bowlby, Ainsworth, and Main and has helped to refine our understanding of how internal working models are formed. It is now recognized that there are significant underpinning neurobiological factors influencing the quality of attachment between the child and caregiver. In fact, given the recent advances, particularly regarding the importance of neurophysiology and neurocircuitry to these processes, we see Sigmund Freud's dreams beginning to be realized. In Freud's early writings, he expressed eagerness for the day when his psychoanalytic concepts could be understood through biological process. Miller and Katz (1989) state "Freud's eventual theories of psychoanalysis rested on his insistence on a topographical approach to the unconscious that was derived from the structural concepts he borrowed from neurology. He thus formed the foundations for his later theories of psychoanalysis when he studied hysteria as a neurologist."

The Shift from One-Person to Two-Person Psychology

Earlier in this chapter we laid the groundwork for distinguishing between one- and two-person psychologies. In the former, symptomatic improvement occurs through remembering the conflicted past parental relationships with the use of free associations, which involve repeating early neurotic maladaptive patterns with the analyst through transference. Once a transference neurosis is apprehended [with help from the analyst's interpretations to make the unconscious conscious: "where id is, there shall ego be" (Freud 1920)], the patient can work through it. During the early 1990s, traditional theorists struggled to openly embrace the emerging theoretical formulations of a two-person psychology. In the psychoanalytic world of the time, two-person psychology was negatively perceived and believed to be a form of "wild analysis" (Schafer 1985). The idea of a two-person, relationally based psychoanalysis and psychotherapy shook the foundations of traditional psychoanalytic theory in positing that the patient's healing would come about with the active presence of the "real person" in the analyst or therapist, who would cocreate a new "corrective emotional experience" (Alexander et al. 1946; Hoffman 1992; Mitchell 2003). Alexander et al coined the term *corrective emotional experience* holding that it is the fundamental therapeutic principle of psychotherapy: "to re-expose the patient, under more favorable circumstances, to emotional situations which he could not handle in the past" (Alexander et al. 1946). They added that "intellectual

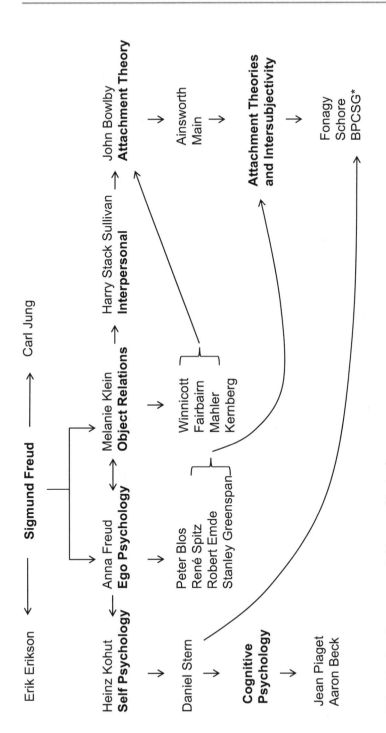

Fig. 2.5 Lineage of psychodynamic theories and theorists

insight alone is not sufficient," a sentiment with which most psychotherapists agree. In short, the patient, in order to be helped, must undergo an engineered, participatory emotional experience to repair the traumatic influence of actual past experiences. This idea was initially dismissed from psychoanalytic circles, and it was not until the1990s that the concept was reintroduced, with two-person psychology theorists recognizing its relevance to psychoanalysis and psychotherapy. Among the leading empirically based psychoanalytic relational theorists over the last 20 years are Stephen Mitchell, Irwin Hoffman, Jessica Benjamin, Lewis Aron, Jay Greenberg, Emmanuel Ghent, Philip Bromberg, Charles Spezzano, Adrienne Harris, Owen Renik, Donnel Stern, Jeremy Holmes, and Paul Wachtel.

The principal neurodevelopmental (and relational) theorists of the past 40 years include René Spitz, Robert Emde, Peter Fonagy, Daniel Stern, and Allan Schore (Fig. 2.5). They all had intimate knowledge of traditional psychoanalytic theories and theoreticians, from which their work derived (Palombo et al. 2012). Among these theorists, René Spitz (1887–1974) was the first to base his research on direct infant observation with video recordings that allowed his research team to carefully analyze the details of interactions and communications between infant and caregiver. Early on, Spitz noted the impact of severe maternal depravation in the failure-to-thrive syndrome in infants (Spitz 1965). Robert Emde (1935–), a student of Spitz, is known for his infant research studies on social referencing, which the caregiver must provide the infant to promote a sense of security to explore and analyze the world: "the self is a social self to begin with" (Emde 2009). Recapitulating this concept, Emde emphasized the importance of the "we-go," a play on the "ego" that had dominated one-person psychology for the half-century prior to Emde's infant studies. The use of his term in the seminal paper "From Ego to 'We-Go': Neurobiology and Questions for Psychoanalysis" underscored that from "infancy, innately given brain processes support social reciprocity and the development of "we-ness"" (Emde 2009).

In a parallel, the British psychologist and psychoanalyst Peter Fonagy (1952–) theorized that infants can learn to regulate internal affective states when the caregiver promotes their capacity to "mentalize" (see mentalization, this Chapter). Later, Allan Schore (1943–), a developmental psychologist, began to formulate a regulatory theory that emphasized the role of the experience-dependent emotional-processing neurocircuitry. His work centers on a relational unconscious that becomes active when the infant's unconscious affective state resonates with the caregiver's experience-dependent maturation of the emotion-processing system, allowing the infant to develop internal working models of the attachment (Schore 2003, 2009). He further believes that these internal working models are stored in non-declarative memory systems in the right cerebral cortex. Similarly, Daniel Stern (1934–2012) is known for his contributions to the emerging concept of *intersubjectivity,* a psychodynamic term that refers to a person's capacity to share and participate in the subjective experience of another. Stern et al liken this phenomenon to "the oxygen we breathe but never see or think of" and emphasizes that the experience of two persons interacting is determined by the here and now, "present moments" within the intersubjective space cocreated by both, a meeting of the minds that create a mutually shared encounter (Stern et al. 1998).

Intersubjectivity and the Exasperated Family of a Psychiatrically-Hospitalized Adolescent

A 12-year-old girl, originally from Honduras, was adopted when she was two by midwestern parents who were both professionals and were happy in their marriage. Her adoptive parents had good cognitive flexibility, easy/flexible temperaments (Chap. 3), a good capacity to mentalize, and a history of secure attachment. Their adoptive daughter was the opposite; she had many explosive and aggressive episodes that at times led the parents to hold her down to prevent her from hurting herself or them. They shared their frustration with medical providers, concerned that their daughter did not show "any remorse" after these violent outbursts. The episodes were increasing in frequency and intensity, with minimal improvement in spite of regular outpatient psychiatric services that included individual, family, and pharmacological therapies. Feeling hopeless about her progress and fearing for their well-being, the adoptive parents had begun to consider calling social services for the removal of their adopted daughter from the home. When she was admitted to her third inpatient psychiatric hospitalization, the parents felt validated, stating, "Medications and therapy do not work on her. She is not fixable." It was immediately apparent to the inpatient psychiatrist, in the first interview, that the child had cognitive deficits as evidenced by her concrete thinking, poor procedural memory, and limited cognitive flexibility in processing emotions. This was confirmed by a full battery of psychological testing. She also presented as having the difficult/feisty temperament style using the criteria set forth by Thomas and Chess (Chap. 3).

Due to her biological mother's active use of illicit drugs during pregnancy, the child had a history of poor prenatal care. Born at 35 weeks, she spent her first 2 years of life in Honduran foster homes. This clearly had a negative influence in her cognitive, psychological, and social-development milestones. At age 10 she had been diagnosed as having an oppositional defiant disorder, reactive attachment disorder, and generalized anxiety disorder.

During an early treatment-team meeting, after the members had met with the patient and family on several occasions, the team social worker expressed a strong empathy for both the child in her limitations and for the parents in their difficulties parenting her. She also shared that "there is something about the parents I don't like. They don't seem to show any empathy toward their daughter when they visit her. They don't give the child any smiles or hugs, so sad." Fortunately, before the treatment-team meeting, the attending child psychiatrist had interviewed the girl in her room. Due to her disruptive behavior, she had been sent to her room from the treatment milieu group. Having knowledge of her cognitive deficits and temperamental difficulties, the child psychiatrist tried to engage her by showing interest in her favorite games and music. During the interview, the intersubjecitve experience the child psychiatrist was co-creating with the patient was very similar to the one the treatment team social worker had described in relation to her parents: "They do not seem to show any empathy." The patient made no effort to connect with the child psychiatrist, in spite of his attempts to play and draw with markers to capitalize on her strengths with visual spatial skills. She refused to participate and withdrew into her angry affective state, blaming the unit staff, with no hint of remorse for disrupting the milieu group. The child psychiatrist's subjective experience was that of wanting to be removed from the interaction to avoid having the feelings of hopelessness about the patient's future. He, like the parents, subjectively felt "What is the point in giving her hugs and smiles?" and noted experiencing sadness that the child was not able to relate to him. The intersubjective experience had been co-created though both the child psychiatrist's wishes to "help" the patient and the patient's inability to mentalize the experience as a corrective one. Her internal regulatory system had neurological deficits which left her unaware that her subjective implicit self was that of a primitive child with minimal reciprocity. She was unable to hold in mind the experience of the other person and was bound to seek gratification of her unregulated needs. The child psychiatrist shared with the treatment team his understanding of the interaction and wondered whether his feelings lent insight into the parents': a sense of hopeless about the future of the child due to her neuro-cognitive deficits, which prevented her from engaging in relationships. The child psychiatrist worked with the nursing staff and psychiatric treatment team to see things from the parents' point of view: 10 years of caring for a difficult child who was unable to provide them with emotional reciprocity and joy. The treatment team agreed and conveyed to the parents that they better grasped their dilemma in caring for their daughter. When the social worker shared in an empathic manner that the treatment team now recognized how they—adoptive parents—must have felt, exhausting themselves by providing affection to a child that had difficulty reciprocating their kindness, the parents, in tears, expressed that they finally felt understood and not blamed.

They openly shared that initially they had felt that the treatment team considered them a bad fit for their child because they did not provide affection to her "in front of the unit staff." They explained that after many years of effort in providing affection to their daughter, they had begun to resent that she was unable to value their love and, still weeping, added, "We now know that it is not her fault. She has neurological deficits."

As this case demonstrates, understanding a person takes more than just listening. The interactions between the patient and members of the treatment team are co-created, shared experience. It is impossible for any person to know in advance how another will relate to them. How the members of a treatment team approach a patient will invariably affect how the patient responds. For example, when treatment-team members approach a patient in a friendly and jovial manner, the patient usually responds similarly. By contrast, if team members approach the patient in a professional and distant manner, the patient will likely feel talked down to, which may evoke implicit memories of early negative experiences, causing the patient to respond in a defensive and distancing manner. This first relational moment will shape the many other moments that are to emerge from their interactions.

Poor social competence that stems from cognitive deficits, temperamental traits, and disorganized attachment schemas will not dissipate with age or educational achievement.

Thus, the psychiatric consultant, like the child psychiatrist described above, will need to keep in mind that his interventions and recommendations will result from the interplay of multiple "subjectivities" that will focus on the "here and now" experiences of all involved parties. In short, intersubjectivity will be forever present in the work with patients, their families, and treatment teams, and the psychiatric consultant, knowingly or unknowingly, will use intersubjectity in guiding his or her recommendations.

Mentalization and Intersubjectivity: Are They Different?

The reader, at this point, may wonder whether there are differences between mentalization and intersubjectivity. We suggest that mentalization-based theories contain aspects of both one-person and two-person psychologies, whereas intersubjectivity is exclusively a two-person psychology. We recognize that both concepts are "theories of mind," and both are relational theories. Regarding mentalization, Allen et al. (2008) note, "the concept of mentalizing first emerged in psychoanalysis: Freud implicitly employed the concept of mentalizing in his initial neurobiological theory of the development of the mind." They later add, "It is no accident that within psychoanalysis, object relations theory has been especially compatible with focusing on mentalzing in treatment." He further clarifies that mentalizing in clinical practice "might be viewed as equidistant between psychodynamic psychotherapy and cognitive therapy." By contrast, Wallin (2007) notes that intersubjectivity "is the permeability or 'interpenetrability' of personal boundaries that allow us to participate in the subjective experience of other people." He adds that intersubjectivity may be "seen as a matter not just of communication but . . . 'interpersonal communion'" (Wallin 2007). The concept of interpersonal communion is best described by Stern: "it is a form of nonmagical mindreading via interpreting overt behaviors such as posture, tone of voice, speech rhythm, and facial expression, as well as verbal content" (Stern 2005). These contemporary controversies are far from over, and we refer the reader to recent reviews that address them (Wachtel 2010). These unique clinical concepts, mentalization, and intersubjectivity will be used when applicable—and not interchangeably—throughout the book when discussing clinical material.

2.4 Summary

In this chapter, we have provided a foundation to better comprehend the importance that innate biological and genetic processes have in forming a patient's unique core sense of self, as well as their intrapsychic and interpersonal psychological functioning. With a greater grasp of these concepts, the consulting psychiatrist can begin to use the psychodynamic tenets to understand the patient's personality style and may develop a psychodynamic formulation, regardless of his or her theoretical orientation, to facilitate the implementation of practical treatment interventions in difficult consultations.

Some readers may feel that this chapter is heavy-handed with psychodynamic theory and not attachment theory, while others may consider there is not sufficient emphasis of classic psychodynamic theory and too much on contemporary attachment theory. It is not our aim in this book to provide an in-depth analysis of the similarities and differences between each very useful theory. Rather, we hope to provide an easy way to employ, in a practical sense, each theory as it pertains to the patient, family, and treatment-team members psychodynamically. When the interaction between patient and others is approached in a psychodynamic way, a balanced framework results—a framework that can be easily explored within the short time period that the consulting psychiatrist or child psychiatrist usually has to devote to his or her cases, whether or not they are difficult consultations. For those wanting a more in-depth study of psychodynamic and attachment theories, we provide references for the detailed review of the interested student.

References

Ainsworth MDS, Blehar M, Waters E et al (1978) Patterns of attachment: a psychological study of the strange situation. Lawrence Erlbaum Associates, Hillsdale NJ, p 37

Akhtar S (2009) Comprehensive dictionary of psychoanalysis. Karnac Books, London

Alexander F, French TM, Bacon CL et al (1946) Psychoanalytic therapy: principles and application. Ronald Press, New York, pp 66–70

Allen JG, Fonagy P (2006) The handbook of mentalization-based treatment, First Edition. Wiley, New York

Allen JG, Fonagy P, Bateman A (2008) Mentalizing in clinical practice. American Psychiatric Publishing, Washington, DC

American Psychiatric Association (2000) Diagnostic and statistical manual of mental disorders. Text Revision. DSM-IV-TR, 4th edn. American Psychiatric Publishing, Washington, DC

American Psychiatric Association (2013) Diagnostic and statistical manual of mental disorders. 5th Edition DSM-5, 5th edn. American Psychiatric Association, Washington, DC

Aron L (1990) One person and two person psychologies and the method of psychoanalysis. Psychoanal Psychol 7:475–485

Bateman A, Fonagy P (2008) 8-year follow-up of patients treated for borderline. Am J Psychiatry 165(5):631–638

Bateman A, Fonagy P (2009) Randomized controlled trial of outpatient mentalization-based treatment versus structured clinical management for borderline. Am J Psychiatry 166 (12):1355–64

Benoit D (2004) Infant-parent attachment: definition, types, antecedents, measurement and outcome. Paediatr Child Health 9(8):541–545

Boston Process and Change Study Group (2010) Change in psychotherapy: a unifying paradigm. WW Norton & Company, New York

Bowlby J (1999) Attachment, 2nd edition, attachment and loss, vol 1. Basic Books, New York

Brenner C (1974) An elementary textbook of psychoanalysis. Random House, New York

Bretherton I (1992) The origins of attachment theory: John Bowlby and Mary Ainsworth. Dev Psychol 28:759–775

Cicirelli VG (1991) Attachment theory in old age: protection of the attached figure. In: Pillemer K, McCartney K (eds) Parent-child relations throughout life. Erlbaum, New Jersey, pp 25–42

Cicirelli VG (1998) Feelings of attachment to siblings and well-being in later life. Psychol Ageing 4:211–216

Delgado SV, Songer D (2009) Personality disorders and behavioral disturbances. In more than medication: incorporating psychotherapy into community psychiatry appointments. Matrix Medical Communications, Edgemont, PA, pp 65–76

Emde RN (2009) From Ego to "We-Go": Neurobiology and questions for psychoanalysis: commentary on papers by Trevarthen, Gallese, and Ammaniti & Trentini. Psychoanal Dial 19:556–564

Fonagy P, Gergely G, Jurist EL et al (2002) Affect regulation, mentalization and the development of the self. Other Press, New York

Freud S (1905) Three essays on the theory of sexuality. In: Strachey J (ed) The standard edition, vol 7. The Hogarth Press, London, pp 130–243

Freud S (1914) Remembering, repeating and working through. In: Strachey J (ed) The, vol 12, Standardth edn. Hogarth Press, London, pp 147–156

Freud S (1916-1917) Introductory lectures on psycho-analysis, part III. The standard edition, vol 16. Hogarth Press, London, pp 441–447

Freud S (1920) Beyond the pleasure principle. In: Strachey J (ed) The standard edition, vol 18. Hogarth Press, London, pp 7–64

Freud S (1924) The dissolution of the Oedipus complex. In: Strachey J (ed) The standard edition, vol 19. Hogarth Press, London, pp 172–179

Freud S (1938) The splitting of the ego in the defensive process, vol 23. Hogarth Press, London, pp 275–278

Freud A (1966) The ego and the mechanisms of defense. Hogarth Press, London, Original work published in 1937

Gabbard GO (2010) Long-term psychodynamic psychotherapy: a basic text. American Psychiatric Publishing, Arlington, VA, pp 151–152

Gabbard GO, Wilkinson SM (1994) Management of countertransference with borderline patients. American Psychiatric Publishing, Washington, DC

Greenberg J (2003) Commentary on psychoanalytic discourse at the turn of our century: a plea for a measure of humility. J Am Psychoanal Assn 51S:89–98

Groves JE (1978) Taking care of the hateful patient. N Engl J Med 298(16):883–887

Hartman H (1958) Ego psychology and the problem of adaptation. (trans: Rapaport D). International Universities Press, New York, First edition published in 1939

Hoffman IZ (1992) Some practical implications of a social-constructivist view of the psychoanalytic situation. Psychoanal Dial 2:287–304

Hooper LM, Tomek S, Newman CR (2011) Using attachment theory in medical settings: implications for primary care physicians. J Ment Health 21(1):23–37

Horwitz L (2005) The capacity to forgive: intrapsychic and developmental perspectives. J Am Psychoanal Assoc 53:485–511

Kernberg OF (1976) Object relations theory and clinical psychoanalysis. Jason Aronson, New York

Kernberg O (2000) Borderline conditions and pathological narcissism. Aronson, New York

Klein M (1932) The psychoanalysis of children. Hogarth Press, London

Kohut H (1971) The analysis of the self: a systematic approach to the psychoanalytic treatment of narcissistic personality disorders. International Universities Press, New York

Laugharne R (2013) Personality disorders in consultation-liaison psychiatry. Curr Opin Psychiatry 26(1):84–89

Main M (2000) Recent studies in attachment: overview, with selected implications for clinical work. In: Goldberg S, Muir R, Kerr J (eds) Attachment theory: social, developmental, and clinical perspectives. Analytic Press, Hillsdale, NJ, pp 407–474

Main M, Goldwyn R (1984) Predicting rejection of her infant from mother's representation of her own experiences: a preliminary report. Child Abuse Negl 8:203–217

Main M, Goldwyn R (1998) Adult attachment scoring and classification system (Manuscript). University of California at Berkeley, Berkeley, CA

Main M, Solomon J (1990) Procedures for identifying infants as disorganized/disoriented during the Ainsworth Strange situation. In: Greenberg MT, Cicchetti D, Cummings EM (eds) Attachment in the preschool years: theory, research, and intervention. University of Chicago Press, Chicago, pp 121–160

Main M, Kaplan N, Cassidy J (1985) Security of infancy, childhood, and adulthood: a move to the level of representation. Monogr Soc Res Child Dev 50(1–2):66–104

Mancia M (2006) Implicit memory and early unrepressed unconscious: their role in the therapeutic process: How the neurosciences can contribute to psychoanalysis. Int J Psychoanal 87:83–103

Masterson JF (2005) The personality disorders through the lens of attachment theory and the neurobiologic development of the self. A clinical integration. Zeig, Tucker & Theisen, New York

Maunder RG, Hunter JJ (2001) Attachment and psychosomatic medicine: developmental contributions to stress and disease. Psychosom Med 63(4):556–567

McLean J (2007) Psychotherapy with a narcissistic patient using Kohut's self-psychology model. Psychiatry (Edgmont) 4(10):40–47

Miller NS, Katz JL (1989) The neurological legacy of psychoanalysis: Freud as a neurologist. Compr Psychiatry 30(2):128–134

Mitchell SA (2003) Relationality: from attachment to intersubjectivity. Routledge, New York

Mitchell SA, Black MJ (1995) Freud and beyond: a history of modern psychoanalytic thought. Basic Books, New York

Palombo J, Bendicsen HK, Koch BJ (2012) Guide to psychoanalytic developmental theories. Springer, New York

Parkes CM, Stevenson-Hinde J, Marris P (1991) Attachment across the lifecycle. Tavistock/ Routledge, London

Renik O (2004) Intersubjectivity in psychoanalysis. Int J Psycho-Anal 85:1053–1056

Rinsley DB (1982) Borderline and other self-disorders. Jason Aronson, New York

Rossouw TI, Fonagy P (2012) Mentalization-based treatment for self-harm in adolescents: a randomized controlled trial. J Am Acad Child Adolesc Psychiatry 51(12):1304–1313

Schafer R (1985) Wild analysis. J Am Psychoanal Assoc 33:275–279

Schore AN (2003) Affect dysregulation and disorders of the self. WW Norton & Company, New York

Schore AN (2009) Relational trauma and the developing right brain: an interface of psychoanalytic self psychology and neuroscience. Ann N Y Acad Sci 1159:189–203

Shaver PR, Hazan C (1988) A biased overview of the study of love. J Soc Pers Relat 5:473–501

Spitz RA (1965) The first year of life: a psychoanalytic study of normal and deviant development of object relations. International Universities Press, New York

Stern DN (2004) The present moment in psychotherapy and everyday life. WW Norton & Company, New York, pp 97–111

Stern DN (2005) Intersubjectivity. In: Person ES, Cooper AM, Gabbard GO (eds) Textbook of psychoanalysis, 1st edn. The American Psychiatric Publishing, Arlington, VA, pp 77–92

Stern DN, Sander LW, Nahum JP (1998) Non-interpretive mechanisms in psychoanalytic therapy: the 'something more' than interpretation. Int J Psycho-Anal 79:903–921

Strous RD, Ulman AM, Kotler M (2006) The hateful patient revisited: relevance for 21st century medicine. Eur J Intern Med 17(6):387–393

Sullivan MD, Ciechanowski PS, Russo JE et al (2009) Understanding why patients delay seeking care for acute coronary syndromes. Circ Cardiovasc Qual Outcomes 2(3):148–154

Vaillant GE (1992) Ego mechanisms of defense: a guide for clinicians and researchers. American Psychiatric Press, Washington, DC

Wachtel PL (2010) One-person and two-person conceptions of attachment and their implications for psychoanalytic thought. Int J Psycho-Anal 91:561–581

Wachtel PL (2011) Therapeutic communication, second edition: knowing what to say when. Guilford Press, New York

Wallin D (2007) Attachment in psychotherapy. Guilford Press, New York, 55

Weiss RS (1982) Attachment in adult life. In: Parkes CM, Stevenson-Hinde J (eds) The place of attachment in human behavior. Basic Books, New York, pp 171–184

Weiss RS (1991) The attachment bond in childhood and adulthood. In: Marris P, Stevenson- Hinde J, Parkes C (eds) Attachment across the life cycle. Routledge, New York, pp 66–76

Winnicott DW (1965) The maturational processes and the facilitating environment. International Universities Press, New York, pp 73–82

The Patient

3

> *You always make each day a special day. By just you're being you. There's only one person exactly like you in the whole world. And that's you yourself*
> —Fred Rogers "Mr. Rogers" (1928–2003)

3.1   From the Inside Out

In the training of psychiatrists who treat adults as well as those who focus on children and adolescents, the empathic doctor–patient relationship is recognized as the foundation upon which all successful treatments are constructed. Establishing rapport with the patient, with mutual respect, facilitates the desired treatment outcomes and, as such, is the *sine qua non* of psychiatric practice. Patients who suffer from mental illness are necessarily asked, when possible, to share the history of their history of present illness with a timeline that establishes when they first noticed their symptoms, the frequency of symptoms, variations in the intensity of symptoms over time, along with precipitating and perpetuating factors. Over the course of the traditional psychiatric evaluation, the clinician may quickly become focused on elucidating risk factors, identifying predictors of treatment response, and determining which "symptoms" meet threshold criteria for a disorder. Thus, with the standard use of the *Diagnostic and Statistical Manual of Mental Disorders 5th Edition* (*DSM-5*, American Psychiatric Association 2013), the diagnosis is based on a collection of signs, and symptoms that have been well defined. Importantly, however, when a diagnosis is based solely on the use of *DSM-5* criteria, critical insight into an effective treatment regimen may be lost. The role of patients within the difficult psychiatric consultation can be determined using information they themselves provide. By inquiring about the patient's life story, which includes experiences that have shaped their personality, with attention to their relationships with family, friends, and coworkers as well as to their accomplishments and hardships, we gain a better understanding of the patient's strengths and weaknesses that will enhance or interfere with treatment efforts. The consulting psychiatrist is

S.V. Delgado and J.R. Strawn, *Difficult Psychiatric Consultations*,
DOI 10.1007/978-3-642-39552-9_3, © Springer-Verlag Berlin Heidelberg 2014

Table 3.1 A comparison of a traditional *DSM-5*-based approach to the patient's history (left) and an approach that includes both *DSM-5* criteria and the patient's life story (right)

The patient is a 17-year-old adolescent with a history of generalized anxiety disorder and social anxiety disorder. At initial outpatient presentation, the patient described persistent fear of social situations, was preoccupied by how his peers perceived him, and avoided most social activities, including school. He had demonstrated limited improvement in school avoidance and withdrawal from social situations, despite ongoing cognitive-behavioral psychotherapy and fluoxetine, which had been titrated to 20 mg daily and reportedly worsened his anxiety. The patient and his mother also described intense concern about his future, a constant sense of inner tension and restlessness, as well as anxious ruminations that were associated with initial and middle insomnia. Moreover, he described recurrent headaches in times of anxiety, and he had recently terminated his part-time employment at a local restaurant.	John is a 17-year-old adolescent who has had severe anxiety since his parents divorced (when he was 11), due to his father's affair with another woman. John struggled with significant anxiety and met *DSM-5* criteria for generalized anxiety disorder and social anxiety disorder. When John and his mother first met the psychiatrist, his mother appeared hesitant in her interactions and seemed untrusting. She explained that since her divorce, it had been "just John and me" and shared that both were close, adding that, "He is totally open about everything with me." John said little and seemed to seek regular reassurance from his mother when asked questions. He gradually began to speak of how he avoided most social situations and instead spent time at home with his mother. During prior treatment with weekly cognitive-behavioral psychotherapy and fluoxetine, provided by their last psychiatrist, the closeness between parent and child, which seemed to be interfering with John's adolescent developmental progress, were not addressed. John expressed worry over his future and described a constant sense of inner tension and restlessness, as well as anxious ruminations that were associated with initial and middle insomnia. He also shared that he feared that something would happen to his mother if he were not available to her. John and his mother were seen on a weekly basis in psychodynamic family therapy, and soon, after his symptoms improved, he began to socialize more and his mother began to encourage John to attend the therapy sessions alone as she was better able to tolerate his steps toward independence. However, given that John continued to experience some residual anxiety, his psychiatrist initiated sertraline monotherapy and titrated the sertraline to 150 mg daily).
Fluoxetine was discontinued, and over 8 weeks, sertraline monotherapy was initiated and titrated to 150 mg daily. Although there was some improvement in his subjective anxiety, he reported persistent social anxiety. Over the following 2 months, the patient experienced a continuing decrease in his anxiety, was less concerned about others' perceptions of him, and was able to attend church and begin applying for a part-time job. He also reported improvement in his anxiety-related insomnia, a decrease in his sense of inner tension and restlessness, and diminished somatic symptoms. Nevertheless, he continued to fear being away from home and avoided social activities with friends.	

The reader will note that the latter approach elucidates the manner in which the patient's symptoms fluctuated with regard to family-system issues and his prior developmental experiences

charged with incorporating the information obtained from the patient, from his or her family, and also other sources (e.g., prior medical or psychiatric treatment records, etc.) into the recommendations for the treatment team, whether they be psychopharmacologic or psychotherapeutic (Table 3.1).

While keeping the *DSM-5* in mind as a resource for the psychiatric consultant, we will review the importance in consultative work of understanding the patient's life story. This understanding should not be limited to a person's psychodynamic aspects; the clinician should also consider the contribution of the patient's innate temperament and social cognition in the formation of their psychodynamic self against the backdrop of the family and of the social and cultural environment in which they have lived. One might describe this approach as a grasp of the interplay between the forces of *nature and nurture*. Although many psychodynamic and attachment-theory texts pay limited attention to cognitive functioning and temperament in forming personality, contemporary research has demonstrated that individual's genetic makeup is a determining factor, and it has also expanded our understanding of the many ways that family, friends, and life events mediate the selection of the experiences stored in what is often referred to as implicit relational memory, which some consider the basis of the psychodynamic self (Mancia 2006). Herein, we will briefly review the manner in which cognitive functioning and temperament can have a profound impact on how a person approaches the life's complexities and, more importantly, how they manage adversity, as in the case of a medical or psychiatric illness. As Sander Koole, PhD, eloquently noted, "Emotion regulation emerges as one of the most far-ranging and influential processes at the interface of cognition and emotion" (Koole 2009).

3.2 Cognitive Functioning

In understanding a patient, it is important to take into account their cognitive abilities, particularly with regard to the norms of their age. In routine practice, clinicians commonly perform a mental-status examination and may write a brief comment about the patient's cognitive function (e.g., fund of knowledge, logical process, etc.). Such a superficial evaluation may be disadvantageous, however, in approaching consultations where parties are at a treatment impasse, as the clinician may remain unaware that core cognitive capacities are the root of the problem. At a minimum, the psychiatric consultant should assess whether the patient has the ability to interpret what their treatment plan involves without major distortions. When in physical or psychological distress, a patient may temporarily be unable to process the many diagnostic results or treatment recommendations. An example: during his colonoscopy, Dr. Adams, a competent internist, becomes overwhelmed when told by his gastroenterologist that he has a "malignant-looking polyp." He returns to work and finds himself forgetting the names of his recently hired nursing staff and is unable to recall the agenda items for his administrative meetings. His mental status would indicate superior intelligence at baseline and currently having difficulties with memory and reasoning due to preoccupation with a possible malignancy in his colon. In contrast, a 25-year-old woman is diagnosed with idiopathic thrombocytopenic purpura, and treatment with corticosteroids is recommended. She is told to avoid activities that could cause injury and to limit her use of alcohol. Her hematologist is surprised at the intense and hostile reaction, as he has shared that her prognosis is very good and that improvement could be expected within a short period of time. Believing that she had been diagnosed with "blood cancer" and was called an "alcoholic," the patient becomes irate and threatens to take legal action against the hematologist. A psychiatric consultation is requested, and it is found that the patient has struggled most her life with a receptive-language disorder that results in her misinterpreting information, though she excels in visual and hands on tasks. The psychiatric consultant asks the hematologist to make use of visual materials to explain the patient's illness in more detail and to draw a timeline describing how the corticosteroids are to be taken and tapered off. The effects of alcohol in slowing the production of platelets are also visually explained. Though the patient's "mental status" may have been reported as of "average intelligence," this reduction fails to capture the receptive-language deficits that would likely place her in the below-average range for reciprocal verbal exchanges. Assessing her cognitive function revealed the way to approach the problem. In short, when one embarks in clinical decision making, it is critical to assess the person's cognitive abilities. Not only can cognitive strengths and weaknesses affect a patient's ability share personal experiences with others, they can also significantly influence the understanding and management of their illness and their interactions with the treatment team. As with Dr. Adams, reasoning can be temporarily impaired due to anxiety about one's own well-being, and "viewing the world as a safe and predictable place and seeing oneself as a competent agent in that world are important psychosocial resources for handling stress" (Turner and Roszell 1994) will allow for use of inner strengths. In extreme cases of bereavement or depression, the patient may present with what appears as severe cognitive deficits and having access to a baseline cognitive evaluation can help the clinician discover and appeal to their innate strengths.

In difficult psychiatric consultations, there are times when the consultant, the family, or the treatment team may request formal cognitive testing. In these cases, families are usually relieved to have concrete evidence of their ailing relative's strengths and limitations, and once they understand the reasons their loved one's experience of the treatment team is repeatedly misinterpreted, their anxieties diminish. Imaging studies have shown structural and functional brain abnormalities associated with the presence of these cognitive and linguistic communication disorders (Delgado et al. 2011; Frodl and Skokauskasm 2012; Lai 2013; Webster et al. 2008). Moreover, by some reports, 10 % of the general population has learning weaknesses, and among this group, many have formal learning disabilities (Altarac and Saroha 2007; Cooper et al. 2007).

Considering these statistics, it is not surprising that learning disorders or learning weaknesses may be frequently observed in difficult psychiatric consultations—not only in the patient, but, as illustrated in the vignette below, also in family members, whose cognitive deficits may prevent them from recognizing the patient's limitations.

The Learning-Disabled Adolescent

A 16-year-old girl is admitted to a general pediatric inpatient unit for the treatment and management of her diabetes. During her stay, she shares with the treatment team that she feels overwhelmed in managing her diabetes and that the day before, while at school, she had suicidal ideation and felt like "just letting go of life." The treatment team requests a psychiatric consultation to assess the patient's safety and to evaluate for possible depression, as they have stabilized her blood sugars and are "ready to discharge her." The treating physician requests that the treatment-team social worker provide the education needed for the patient and mother to manage the diabetes at home. As the psychiatric consultant completes the evaluation of the patient and her mother, the treatment-team social worker arrives and proceeds to explain, to the patient and her mother, the complexities of diabetes management, the ramifications of poorly controlled blood sugars, and the need for careful monitoring of her blood sugars. Thereafter, the social worker asks the adolescent if she is willing to assume responsibility in managing her diabetes and also asks her mother if she is willing to help her daughter follow through with the recommendations. The psychiatric consultant is not surprised when the patient and her mother readily agree to accept responsibility. They had shared with the consultant that they usually are agreeable to recommendations made by doctors, "even though sometimes we have trouble understanding them." They both fear being seen as difficult if they raise any questions or ask for information to be repeated. However, the patient had previously revealed to the consulting psychiatrist that, upon entering high school, "things got worse. I couldn't remember any of the details about my assignments. I failed math, and I just didn't understand what the teachers said unless I could write it down." Her mother, in tears, had shared that when she was an adolescent it was confirmed that she had a learning disorder, that she "barely made it through high school" and had recently begun attending a technical college that provided tutoring in math and a scribe to help her with classroom work. She was hoping to have her daughter formally tested at school "for a learning problem," saying, "She is just like me, poor kid." Upon probing further, the consulting psychiatrist found that patient had struggled for some time with her learning difficulties, though with the help of her supportive family, she felt that "I really am not a quitter, I just need help. I don't pay attention because I can't understand." With this in mind, the psychiatric consultant—noting that the treatment-team social worker was delivering all her recommendations verbally—intervened, explaining to the social worker that the patient and her mother were withholding their problems with memory and verbal comprehension in order be perceived as a pleasant and compliant family, and that although they both were "willing," they were not "able" to assume full responsibility with the recommendations made. Making the social worker aware of the patient and mother's learning problems, he asked for the recommendations to be delivered in writing to help the family. The social worker's response that "We have never approached matters this way" is discouraging in that it suggests the limited attention generally given to cognitive skills, and this may explain the frequent issues of non-compliance in adolescent diabetes clinics.

Cognitive and Affective Flexibility

As part of any evaluation of a patient's cognitive function, the capacity for cognitive and affective flexibility, also referred to as social cognition, should be assessed. Cognitive and affective flexibility are the aspects of cognition that allow the individual to psychologically approach situations with a degree of openness about the fact that their experience is influenced by another person's state of mind and by the contextual, social, and culturally appropriate norms, and to tolerate some degree of uncertainty.

Cognitive and affective flexibility involve several components: executive function, attention, working memory, and emotion regulation (Johnson 2009; Schmeichel et al. 2008). A child reacts with glee as he or she infers that it is acceptable to play with the toys in the physician's office because they are available in an open bin. An adult is disappointed and understands his or her sports team lost when seeing the scoreboard. Moreover, when a person initially refuses to take medications, they implicitly understand the societal disapproval—family member or physician—even if not present, and the negative medical consequences and proceeds to take the medication. Cognitive and affective flexibility precede the development of language skills which typically emerge from 2 to 5 years of age (Blackwell et al. 2009). Cognitive and affective flexibility permit persons to expand awareness and to accept multiple solutions to novel or unpredictable events. Thus, when there is limited cognitive and affective flexibility, a patient may have less adaptability and less interest in engaging with his or her treatment team. In such a situation, the patient may view the treatment team as interfering with his or her life, may minimize the seriousness of his or her illness and may have difficulties with compliance.

Assessing cognitive and affective flexibility can be done briefly during the routine evaluation. When patients are frightened about their well-being due to a medical or psychiatric illness, the clinician can ease their minds and build rapport by spending a brief amount of time asking a few personal questions, reassuring the patient that they are viewed as a whole person and not as a diagnostic entity. In the course of this exchange, the consultant, in an effort to assess cognitive and affective flexibility, may ask the patient to share their view of themselves, their life achievements and accomplishments, and the importance of their relationship to their spouse, children, and friends before the illness was diagnosed. The interview is intended not to minimize the complexities of the illness but rather to understand the impact it will likely have on the patient and their family system and whether the system will be able to psychologically and cognitively comply with the treatment-team recommendations.

Brief Assessment of Cognitive and Affective Flexibly in Adults

- History of the patient's view of himself before the illness was diagnosed.
- History of the patient's achievements and accomplishments.

- History of the patient's preferred activities with others, including spouse, children, and friends.
- Discussion of how the treatment team can best respond to the patient's emotional needs (e.g., a post-rounding "check in" with the patient and/or family, allowing family or colleagues to visit the patient after "visiting hours").

Cognitive and Affective Flexibility in Adolescents

For a medical or psychiatric illness in an adolescent, the diagnosis and recommended treatment are often shared simultaneously with the patient and his or her parents. In spite of their normal developmental fears and worries about their well-being, adolescents should be allowed to be active participants regarding their need for more information about their illness and the course of action concerning it. How the psychiatric consultant can best help the treatment team communicate with adolescents will depend on the patient's level of cognition and cognitive and affective flexibility. Assessment in adolescents is less complex than with younger children, in that developmentally adolescents begin to have capacities similar to that of adults in understanding the nature of their illness, and their reactions are less influenced by fantasy. It is important to keep in mind that some adolescents respond better to the treatment team when humor is used to engage with them before providing information about their illness. In the example later in this chapter, Jason is comfortable with closeness and uses healthy defense mechanisms (humor, sublimation) that the psychiatric consultant notices and employs to establish an alliance. This allows Jason to later jovially ask the consultant to accompany him to the hospital cafeteria for lunch to discuss his ambivalence in continuing with his chemotherapy. In contrast, other adolescents may prefer a professional, intellectual demeanor. This serious approach allows some adolescents to use isolation of affect and, at times, periods of denial regarding the severity of their illness, which may help them comply with treatment recommendations and improve outcome. The psychiatric consultant should be prepared to encourage the treatment-team leader, who may not be the right personality "fit" for a given patient, to recognize that the information may be best received if delivered by a different team member (e.g., a resident or nurse) with experience in working psychologically with adolescents. This presents the psychiatric consultant with an opportunity for a *teachable moment* that will educate the treatment team in the developmentally different cognitive and emotional abilities of adolescents (Bleiberg 2000; Steinberg 2005).

Brief Assessment of Cognitive and Affective Flexibility in Adolescents

- History of the patient's preferred activities with others including parents, friends, and dating.
- History of the patient's birthday celebrations, favorite persons that attended, and gifts received.

- Review of achievements and accomplishments they feel proud of.
- History of favorite video games, music, and sports activities.
- Discussion with the patient of how the treatment team can best respond to their emotional needs (e.g., a post-rounding "check in" with the patient and/or family, allowing peers to visit the adolescent patient after "visiting hours.")

Cognitive and Affective Flexibility in Preschool and School-Age Children

The diagnosis and treatment of a medical or psychiatric illness in preschool and school-age children is commonly shared with the parents but not with the child, as it is often considered to be overwhelming for them. Despite the belief that informing the child may lead to many fears and worries, some young children are interested in knowing about the implications their diagnosis and treatment plan will have on age-appropriate activities: playing, reading, etc. As with any patient, particularly children, there is no one-size-fits-all approach. Communication with any child should depend on his or her level of cognition as well as his or her cognitive and affective flexibility. The assessment of these in preschool and school-age children is complex in that it needs to take into account the norms of their developmental stages, with input from their parents or caregivers to corroborate their responses, and involves a review of any cognitive delays that may have been present before the medical or psychiatric illness. The responses given by preschool and school-age children can be colored by healthy fantasy, and may be exaggerated due to the stress of illness. Ascertaining the extent of a child's understanding of their illness is critical so that the treatment team can learn to explain the diagnosis and its treatment *at his or her level*. When being told about their illness, some children will respond better with the use of drawings, and some may prefer an intellectual approach and welcome the use of written materials. The treatment team may have members better able to *go to the child's level*, and careful delegation of who will communicate the information can reduce anxiety in young patients, thereby facilitating cooperation with procedures and compliance with treatment. The psychiatric consultant may also need to help the treatment-team leader recognize that another team member—such as a resident or nurse, someone with natural abilities in working psychologically with young children—will be better able to communicate with the patient without causing undue stress. This provides the psychiatric consultant an opportunity for a *teachable moment*, in which the treatment team learns about the developmentally different cognitive and emotional abilities of young children. For young and anxious children, treatment teams should strongly consider involving the patient's parents in the delivery aspects of the treatment plans, if they are not also overwhelmed by their own anxiety. In many cases, parents can serve as caring conduits for their child.

   In working with children, and at times adolescents, the consulting psychiatrist may utilize a "time-tried" projective technique often referred to as the "three wishes scenario." In this frequently employed technique, children are asked to imagine they find a magic genie's lamp, from which they release a genie who will grant them three wishes. The children are encouraged to request whatever they hope for. In using this technique, the clinician can assess defense styles, cognitive and affective flexibility, and avoid the anxiety produced by direct questioning. Importantly, this exercise in consultation work is not intended to be used clinically to develop a hypothesis regarding the psychological meaning of the three wishes as would be in a psychotherapeutic process. The patient's responses may be concrete and limited, indicating the impoverished age-related fantasy life of a child who is likely to fear and misinterpret treatment and will need a great deal of reassurance. By contrast, when the answers and approach to the scenario reflect rich and healthy fantasies—wish for good response to treatment, to return home, etc.—the child will likely be engaged in their recovery process and aware of what is needed of them. In addition, the child's responses to all three wishes should be assessed within the context of their family situation. As an example, a consulting psychiatrist evaluating a 10-year-old girl admitted to the neurology service for *status migranosis* (intractable headaches) inquires as to the girl's "three wishes." The patient describes her wish for the headaches to be gone, for her family to be happy, and, with playful affect, for a new Smartphone with unlimited texting. Her wishes reflect underlying healthy defense mechanisms, caring and concern for her family, and her ability to see herself as integrated within an age-appropriate, stable environment. By contrast, a 10-year-old girl with limited cognitive and affective flexibility who is admitted under the same circumstances may wish "to be on a TV show, to have all the video games in the world," and then with some hesitation adds, "I want to go home." These wishes reveal a limited understanding of her role within the context of her larger world and a perception that the illness is foreign to her "everyday self."

Brief Assessment of Cognitive Flexibility in Preschool and School-Age Children

- Elicit the child's recollection of prior birthday parties and favorite gifts received.
- Ask who the child enjoyed having attend the birthday parties.
- Review the child's achievements and accomplishments as well as other experiences that have made him or her feel proud.
- Obtain a history of their favorite toys, games, video games, and movies.
- Use the common "projective technique" of asking the child, "What would you ask for if a genie granted you three wishes?"

3.3   Temperament

Temperament refers to the "stable moods and behavior profiles observed in infancy and early childhood." Though its first description can be found in Ancient Greece two millennia ago (Kagan 1994), temperament came to the forefront in

developmental psychology and child psychiatry in the 1960s and 1970s (Thomas
and Chess 1977). The relevance that temperament styles have in consultation-
liaison work is multifaceted. Although there have been many classification
schemes, Thomas and Chess (1999) are recognized for their landmark scientific
contribution to the study of temperament. Their seminal work has achieved general
consensus in that its expression has been consistent across situations and over time.
In their study, Thomas and Chess longitudinally evaluated 141 children over 22
years, from early childhood until early adulthood (1982, 1986). Over the course of
this evaluation, nine temperament traits became apparent and are described in more
detail later in this chapter.

Temperament Traits Derived from Thomas et al. (1970)

• Activity level
• Rhythmicity or regularity
• Approach or withdrawal responses
• Adaptability to change
• Sensory threshold
• Intensity of reactions
• Mood
• Distractibility
• Persistence when faced with obstacles

The work of Thomas and Chess confirmed what the British psychoanalyst and
father of attachment theory John Bowlby, MD, (1907–1990) had hypothesized: a
child's temperament influences how the child is experienced by their parents and
significantly shapes how the parents interact with the child (Bowlby 1999). This
way of thinking, where an active and bidirectional relationship exists between the
child and caregiver, represented a significant point of divergence from the previously accepted understanding of the infant as a passive recipient and product of his
or her environment (Mahler et al. 1973). In essence, the child began to be seen as a
full contributor to the "goodness of fit" (Thomas and Chess 1999) between the child
and the parents or caregivers. The two researchers found that "some children with
severe psychological problems had a family upbringing that did not differ essentially from the environment of other children who developed no severe problems,"
and later added that "domineering authoritarian handling by the parents might make
one youngster anxious and submissive and another defiant and antagonistic." Thus,
"theory and practice of psychiatry must take into full account the individual and his
uniqueness" (Thomas et al. 1970). Furthermore, it is important to note that temperament in infancy and early childhood is influenced not only by heredity but also by
environmental experiences (Emde and Hewitt 2001), and as a consequence, temperament is recognized as pivotal to our current understanding of attachment theory
(Chap. 2).

A review of the literature regarding child-temperament reveals that much research has evolved in developmental psychology since the early work of Thomas and Chess, 30 years ago, although some controversies reamin (Zentner and Bates 2008). The works of Kagan (2008), children's behavioral inhibition to the unfamiliar, Rothbart and Bates (2006) temperament classification, and Huizink's (2008) biological make-up, have all provided advances in this complex research arena. In essence, the matter of temperament has many facets; genes, neurobiology, observable behavior patterns of interaction and culture.

In Thomas and Chess' New York Longitudinal Study (Chess et al. 1960), youth who had been evaluated earlier in life were reevaluated at an 18–22-year follow-up ($n = 141$), and a high correlation of childhood temperament with temperament in adulthood was observed, even after taking into account the many variables expected over such a long follow-up interval. Nonetheless, the authors caution that "an ever-present danger, of course, is creating self-fulfilling prophecies" (Thomas and Chess 1999). Thus, it is important to note that despite individual differences in the expression of emotion, motor activity, reactivity, and self-regulation, which are agreed to be genetically and biologically based and are stable central features of temperament (Thomas and Chess 1999), the expression of the temperamental styles can be modified by environmental factors such as the parents' emotional response to their child. Further, most individuals have the capacity to vary in the expression of their temperament traits, although over time one trait will usually dominate the manner in which they approach social situations. The individual's capacity to interact with others in an acceptable manner is greatly determined by the how their environment influences matters of reciprocity according to their own unique temperament styles. Additionally, as temperament is shaped by interactions with others, "its regulation is culturally dependent" (Paulussen-Hoogeboom et al. 2007, Chap. 7).

As mentioned above, temperament traits in childhood highly correlate with those present after the transition to adulthood (Thomas and Chess 1986). A child's temperament and their adult personality share remarkably similar features not only in how they navigate day-to-day interactions with others but also how they manage affect-laden emotional interactions. While temperament and personality are interrelated, they are not one and the same. The former refers to the genetically and biologically based innate behavioral style, while the latter describes how emotions, ego function (Chap. 2), and defense mechanisms (Chap. 2) manifest in an individual with a particular temperament. Although it has been long recognized that temperament has a biological basis, it is the influences present in a person's environment that trigger which traits become more adaptive than others.

Below we provide a brief review of the nine temperament traits based on a classification scheme developed by Herbert Birch, a member of the Thomas and Chess research team. This will be followed in subsequent sections by examples of how these nine traits may present in patients, families, or treatment-team members in difficult psychiatric consultations. These examples serve to illustrate that the traits described do not stand alone in the development of a person's temperament style; rather, they influence one another and define an individual's temperament style in different situations.

Temperament Traits

Activity Level

Activity level is rated as "high" or "low" and reflects whether a person has a tendency to usually be "on the go" or whether they prefer a slower pace, taking a "wait and see" approach to novel interests. A "go-getter" patient who has been a high achiever in daily life can be active in learning the risks and benefits and participate with the treatment team's recommendations for their care. The less active and calm patient may become overly thoughtful and not be able to decide, within a reasonable amount of time, about the treatment recommendation needing prompt intervention.

Distractibility

This trait, generally rated as "distractible" or "not distractible," refers to the degree of concentration and attention given when embarking on a tedious task or the ability to study or work on team projects without being sidetracked. When possible in consultation-liaison work, it is good to establish the patient's baseline attentional capacity and distractibility before the diagnosis, as afterward the individual will be dealing with the anxieties and the narcissistic injury of being ill, which may interfere with their ability to make decisions about the treatment of their illness.

Intensity

This characteristic, described as "intense" or "mild," refers to the strength of the patient's emotional response to novel events, whether positive or negative. The response to new medical information may be handled with intensity and pressure in wanting to go ahead with treatment recommendations with minimal attention to the potential risks or in an upsetting manner with strong display of negative affect and avoidance of following through with the recommendations.

Rhythmicity

This trait is rated as "regular" or "irregular" and refers to the predictability of biological functions like appetite and sleep. Adults with good sense of rhythmicity learn to adapt when faced with frequent early morning bedside rounding visits from their treatment team when in the hospital. As family members, they also adapt well to unusual hours needed to participate in the medical and psychiatric care of a hospitalized loved one.

Sensory Threshold

This aspect of temperament is related to the sensitivity a person has to physical stimuli and is rated as "low" or "high." The rating reflects how a patient may react (positively or negatively) to particular sounds when undergoing magnetic resonance imaging or other loud procedures as well as invasive or painful tests (e.g., electromyography, nerve-conduction studies, etc.). It is helpful to know if the patient has a history of being highly sensitive to noises, lights, and particular types of clothing, as this can alter the receptivity to treatment while in hospital and may be interpreted by treatment team as "the patient is being difficult."

Approach/Withdrawal
This aspect of temperament, like the others, is observed early in life and refers to the child's "typical response to unfamiliar people, objects, and situations and the extremes of this dimension define two categories of children called behaviorally inhibited and uninhibited" (Schwartz et al 2003). Youth with inhibited temperament are more likely to be timid with novel interactions, places, and situations. By contrast, uninhibited children may spontaneously approach these stimuli. With regard to the psychiatric consultation, this dimension will reflect the way in which a patient demonstrates the capacity to participate actively and in collaboration with a treatment team in the decision-making process. Some patients may react with hesitation, and in doing so withdraw, while others may approach the novel provider or situation with interest and be easily able to engage in medical decision making.

Adaptability
Adaptability may be thought of as part of a continuum with approach/withdrawal traits and is rated as adaptive or not adaptive. The patient who is adaptive will likely collaborate actively with the treatment team in reviewing the risks and benefits of treatment approaches and is comfortable with the options available.

Persistence
Persistence is rated as "long" or "short." This trait refers to the length of time a patient takes when asked to participate in the decision-making process in the face of adversity. The patient that rates long in persistence may engage in lengthy discussion about risks and benefits, and over time may be experienced as stubborn and difficult. The patient that rates short may quickly realize his or her need for help from others and promptly agree with treatment recommendations without questioning. There seem to be some common elements of persistence that overlap with the trait of intensity.

Mood
Generally, mood is rated as "positive" or "negative," and in consultation work it refers to the emotional response patients have when difficult medical information is delivered to them. If the patient has the capacity to respond positively, this signifies a realistic outlook about their future. Certain patients temperamentally respond in a negative mood, and it is helpful to clarify if this is typical or if the negativity is new and related to the seriousness of the illness.

Temperament Styles

Thomas and Chess defined three general types of temperament styles, 45 % were classified as "easy or flexible," 15 % "slow-to-warm-up," 10 % as "difficult or feisty," and 35 % as "mixed," a combination of the three (Thomas and Chess 1999).

When recognized, certain clusters of temperament traits can be predictive. In a given situation, for example, the combination of negative mood, high intensity, irregularity, and slow adaptability might define a "difficult" child or adult who is likely to have and cause problems during their life, whereas the cluster of positive mood, positive approach, and high adaptability usually signifies a successful child or adult. While this may not seem surprising, the knowledge of these temperament styles may guide psychiatric consultants in creating practical interventions, and it may also help treatment teams have realistic expectations that are based on an understanding of how genetic and biological factors contribute to the variability of a patient's psychological responses. Temperament schema can aid the consulting psychiatrist in teaching treatment-team members not to identify patients as *difficult and with borderline pathology*, avoiding further interaction with them and requesting the consulting psychiatrist *to "convince them to agree with our recommendations or we will need to discharge them from our care."* Sadly, this impasse has been all too common in academic and hospital settings (Chap. 2). Recognizing and working with a given person's temperament style can improve outcomes of patient, and family, as well as treatment-team interactions.

The Easy or Flexible Temperament Style

This style was found to be present in approximately 45 % of the children studied by Thomas and Chess (1999). The person with an *easy or flexible temperament style* typically has a history of being happy overall and not easily upset by negative news or events. In the case of a patient, this individual typically can transition, with a display of healthy and mild forms of anxiety, from conflicted situations to a positive stance and engage in a cooperative approach to the discussion of difficult treatment interventions. The treatment team of patients with overly flexible characteristics would benefit from not taking their complacency as agreement with treatment. Allowing for opportunities to reassure the patient that is important for the team to know what they are thinking and feeling regarding the recommendations given. Unlike the patient with healthy flexibility that seeks new information from the treatment team, the overly complacent patient will need frequent updates about the status of their health. It is reasonable to allow time for dialogue about their treatment, particularly if the patient sees different attending physicians or residents daily and may be withholding information about their inner state. Their complacency during their hospitalization may not bode well for the need to continue with post-discharge follow-up treatment recommendations as they may require active communication with medical providers.

The Slow-to-Warm-up Temperament Style

The patient with a slow-to-warm-up temperament style (15 %) can quickly withdraw when faced with new and difficult situations that involve complex issues with some degree of uncertainty. Children, adolescents, and adults who present with anxiety and shyness may not have the temperamental style conducive to listening to or understanding the information delivered by the treatment team. These patients may rely on their family members to interact with the treatment team and to make decisions for them, and this may frustrate treatment-team members accustomed to interacting with their patients directly. It is best to attempt to accept the patient's slow-to-warm-up temperament style. In approaching such a "difficult consultation," the consulting psychiatrist may work with the treatment team to help them tolerate working indirectly with the patient through his or her family. However, we recognize that this approach may raise the hackles of some hospital-based medical providers, who are less accustomed to and sometimes uncomfortable working this way.

The Difficult or Feisty Temperament Style

The patient with the difficult or feisty style (10 %) is often reluctant to interact with new people or to venture into new situations. This quality is frequently encountered in patients who have to wait to be seen by the treatment team in the hospital. They perceive the situation as one in which they are not important to the treatment team, even if the team has reasonable explanation for the delay. This usually parallels the negative reactions observed with the nursing staff when they're later than usual taking daily vital signs, drawing labs, or changing dressings. These patients are difficult and create distance with members of the treatment team.

The Mixed Temperament Style

This style of temperament was observed in 35 % of subjects by Thomas and Chess (1982), and, as the name implies, reflects that these individuals utilized a mixture of the nine temperament traits that did not allow for a classification into one of the three groups. Patients who fall into this category are best understood psychologically by the consulting psychiatrist with a detailed assessment of their cognitive functioning as described earlier in this chapter and through inquiry about their personality type and attachment style (Chap. 2).

Temperament in the Context of the Difficult Psychiatric Consultation

Understanding the temperament of a patient and of their family members is of great help to the consulting psychiatrist when reviewing the reasons for the consultation, particularly with regard to difficult psychiatric consultations. It is likely that the consultation request relates to an impasse between members of the larger treatment system: the patient, family, and treatment team. The consultant working with complex clinical consultations may first want to have an understanding of the temperament styles of the active participants in the treatment decision-making process. This will help predict the reaction of a patient to a new and stressful event, like the diagnosis of a serious illness; it provides insight as to why some of the members of a treatment team have difficulty interacting with patient and family, and it informs the consulting psychiatrist how to best intervene, addressing the different reactions observed in the system and developing a practical solution that can be accepted and implemented to diffuse the impasse at hand.

A patient with a difficult/feisty temperament is very similar to a patient with a personality disorder (Chap. 2), or to one with a history of having a disorganized, insecure attachment style. Thus, the psychiatric consultant would benefit from a familiarity with styles of temperament, cognitive and affective flexibility, and attachment styles so as to be able to wear multiple hats, enabling the clinician to effectively understand the patient and provide recommendations that integrate these important aspects.

A Closer Look at How Temperament Styles Impact Inpatient Treatment

Temperament Style in the Hospitalized Child

Though the age of a child has bearing on the developmental issues that need to be taken into account to determine the appropriateness of their reactions to illness, matters are further complicated by the child's temperament. This is influenced by the environment in which he or she lives, which also contributes to the characteristics of the child's attachment style (Chap. 2). A child who presents with a difficult/feisty temperamental style, who lives with parents that have easy/flexible or slow-to-warm-up temperament styles and a history of providing secure attachment to their children, will likely be described by the parents as "*not being happy even when we bend over backwards to make him/her happy*." The parents will speak of their own sense of frustration when trying to reassure and calm their child, which is reflective of the child's matters with goodness of fit, intersubjectivity, cognitive and affective flexibility, and temperament.

By contrast, a child with a difficult/feisty temperament style, whose parents have similar temperaments and who has an insecure attachment style when relating to others, is likely to be experienced by the parents in two distinct ways. While they may feel their child is at times "loving and playful," the parents may lack the ability conceptualize their child as a whole object (see splitting, Chap. 2) and characterize their offspring as "difficult and ungrateful." Such parents may have provided limited comfort to the child earlier in their life, and in doing so may have facilitated a pattern of mistrust with frequent use of immature defense mechanisms, the precursors of a borderline level of organization. We emphasize this aspect to reiterate that temperament style and social cognition are two of the precursors of the attachment pattern the child will develop and perpetuate when becoming a parent.

When children require medical or psychiatric treatment, the patient may be quite frightened and scared about being examined by "doctors." The child with difficult/feisty temperament style frequently makes comments that create complex treatment situations for the treatment team. Such a child may behave poorly toward the hospital staff and make statements like "I am not going to cooperate; I'm not taking that medication; I hate the doctors." The psychiatric consultant, approaching this child, will need to determine the degree to which observed difficult/feisty temperament style is typical (through a history obtained from his or her parents or caregivers), or if this observed temperament reflects a change as a result of the child's fear and anxiety attributable to the hospitalization, the diagnosis, or treatment. If it is a change, the consultant can be of great help by suggesting interventions designed to return the child to the healthier temperament style that existed before.

Temperament Style in the Hospitalized Adolescent

Adolescence is typically described as a difficult period, as it requires a transition from childhood to adulthood with physical, hormonal, and cognitive changes (Delgado 2012). Therefore, the adolescent patient requires careful assessment as to whether the emotional reaction to the diagnosis of a medical or psychiatric illness is based on their temperament style, attachment style, or personality style. Adolescents, like younger children, may also be quite frightened as they find themselves in a stage of their life were the future is uncertain. Careful consideration of collateral information from parents, siblings, or peers is valuable.

Temperament Style in the Hospitalized Adult

Adults with difficult/feisty temperament style are known to consistently have trouble allowing emotional and cognitive reciprocity with others. Collateral information is needed to assess whether the difficult/feisty temperament is new, as in the example with Mr. Green this Chapter, or if it has been a persistent style.

Temperament Style in the Hospitalized Geriatric Patient

The geriatric population has received little attention in regard to temperament-based research. However, among older patients, shifts in temperament should be noted by the consulting psychiatrist and attended to in the consultant's interventions. In addition to shifts in observed temperament style or personality, there are many other issues that are important to address (or at least to be aware of). Specifically, geriatric patients may be coping with normal physical changes and changes in cognitive function, deteriorating physical health, and phase-of-life changes in terms of family and occupational roles. It is best to work collaboratively with the patient's family to ascertain the patient's emotional and psychological functioning at baseline, in the context of their psychosocial environment. The general psychiatric consultant may also wish to enlist the assistance of a geriatric psychiatrist in consultations with older patients.

The Healthy Patient Who Deteriorates Psychologically Following a Diagnosis

Mr. Green, a 58-year-old entrepreneur with a testicular seminoma that has metastasized to his lungs and retroperitoneal lymph nodes, is receiving chemotherapy. Over the course of serial treatments he develops increasing irritability with his family and the oncology treatment team. As time passes, his irritability progressively interferes with his daily interactions with his family. Also, during scheduled visits to the hospital for his chemotherapy treatments, he has difficulties in his interactions with the oncology nursing staff. Following his orchiectomy and lymph-node dissection and early in his course of chemotherapy, his oncologist met with both Mr. Green and his family to discuss his concern about Mr. Green's being resistant to the nurse's efforts to deliver his chemotherapy and asked if the treatment team could request a psychiatric consultation. Surprisingly, Mr. Green agreed, as he also had been bothered by the changes in his personality, saying, "My family and friends are unhappy with me." For the initial consultation, the psychiatric consultant met only with Mr. Green, focusing on the degree to which his symptoms interfered with family functioning. Later, with Mr. Green's consent, the psychiatric consultant met with the family to gather information about possible causes of the patient's irritability. In these discussions, Mr. Green was described by his wife as having been a loving husband and a caring father. He was well respected at work, admired for his prowess at complicated negotiations, and had many close friends. Prior to the diagnosis of the testicular seminoma, which was found during a routine physical examination 3 months prior to the consultation, he was active and enjoyed exercising, traveling, hiking, and spending weekends with family and friends. Although Mr. Green reported being devastated by the initial diagnosis, he quickly "regrouped" and recognized his prognosis was relatively good. As he began treatment, he started experiencing complications from the chemotherapy (including recurrent neutropenic fever), for which he required several brief hospitalizations. Experiencing genuine fear, he recognized his need for emotional support from his wife, children, and colleagues, though he had difficulty openly sharing his need for their help. During the same period, his aging mother became ill and, within several weeks, died from complications of pneumonia. Overwhelmed, Mr. Green became conflicted about continuing chemotherapy. The psychiatric consultant sensitively questioned Mr. Green about what had led him to consider discontinuing his treatment and also gently inquired as to what aspect of it frightened him. The patient began to cry and revealed that he worried constantly about how the medications would affect him. He further shared that 3 years earlier, his father had passed away, and he felt that the treatment team charged with his father's care "wasn't attentive. They made decisions without consulting me. My father deteriorated quickly, and I felt I should have fought against the use of those medications." Mr. Green believed the medications had contributed to his father's death and confessed to constant worry over whether they would affect him the same way. Moreover, Mr. Green felt the need to hide his emotions from his family so that if he passed, they could remember him as a strong man. He believed he was expected to show emotional strength regarding the death of his mother and to not speak of his fear regarding the possibility of his own death, so as to serve as an "example" for his grown children and grandchildren. He hoped his fortitude would help his children cope with the loss of their grandmother. Yet while Mr. Green believed he was demonstrating strength to his family, he had become increasingly angry and irritable, failing to recognize that his emotions were the result of his struggles in confronting his mortality, something accentuated by the recent deaths of his own parents.

Feeling paralyzed by his irritability and anger toward them, the family was also silently angry at Mr. Green for not cooperating with his urologist and oncologist. Additionally, family members had started distancing themselves from both him and his wife, wondering, along with his urologist and oncologist, if they should be prepared for his death. He had sometimes refused to allow the nursing staff to initiate his chemotherapy infusions, and his family began to fear "being without him."

As is demonstrated in Mr. Green's case, when a patient presents in an uncharacteristic manner with regard to ego function, personality, and interactions with family, a difficult psychiatric consultation should ensue. Such consultations should not be evaluated through the lens of a patient "resisting treatment because of irrational fears or psychopathology." In such instances, it is imperative to recognize that the patient's reactions to a medical or psychiatric illness invariably will reverberate through the larger system—family and treatment-team members. Moreover, the fact that Mr. Green's post-diagnosis temperament (i.e., difficult/feisty) contrasts sharply with his pre-diagnosis temperament (i.e., easy/flexible), indicates that interventions should focus on increasing self-reflective function with regard to this dramatic change (Table 3.2).

It became apparent that what his family, urologist, and oncologist believed to be obvious—that is, Mr. Green's diagnosis of testicular seminoma and the sudden death of his mother had led to his irritability—was partially correct. However, the psychiatric consultant was able to intervene in a way that allowed the feelings about the death of his father, which had been reawakened, to surface.

Specifically in this case, the psychiatric consultant posed the question to Mr. Green, "How would we have gotten along before 'all of this happened?'" In asking this, the consultant was able to create an emotional space in which Mr. Green could safely explore the shift in his temperament that occurred after his diagnosis.

Diagnostic Formulation and Interventions for Mr. Green (Table 3.2). *The Patient.* Following his diagnosis of testicular seminoma, Mr. Green demonstrates his cognitive and affective flexibility in his interactions with others, but the anxiety related to his illness and the recent deaths of his parents leads to significant psychological changes. In short, a shift occurs in his observed temperament style, from easy/flexible to a difficult/feisty. Accompanying the

Table 3.2 Mr. Green, a healthy executive who temporarily experiences a psychological deterioration following a devastating diagnosis

	Patient before diagnosis	Patient after diagnosis	Family before diagnosis	Family after diagnosis	Treatment team members	Suggested consultant's intervention
Observed cognition	Flexible		Flexible		Flexible	• Given that both the patient and his family have flexible cognition, supportive psychodynamic intervention is appropriate
Observed temperament	Easy/flexible	*Difficult/ feisty*	Easy/flexible		Easy/flexible	• After noting that the temperament of the family and treatment team remains stable, the consultant focuses on the shift in the patient's observed temperament, defense mechanisms, attachment style, and role within the family. The consultant initially "joins" Mr. Green and facilitates sharing the anger and frustrations related to having a serious illness
Observed defense mechanisms	Altruism Sublimation Humor	*Denial Suppression Displacement*				• The consultant helps Mr. Green remember times in which he was admired by his family for his easy/flexible temperament
Observed attachment style	Secure	*Dismissive*	Secure		Secure	• The consultant supports the transition from observed relational patterns to his previously adaptive patterns
Family	Stabilizer	*Scapegoat*	Stabilizer			• The consultant engages Mr. Green, discussing his worries openly with family and treatment team
						• The consultant reframes the role Mr. Green's wife and adult children need to take in order to support him during the course of treatment

The table may be used to succinctly identify and assess the areas that require action by the psychiatric consultant in complex psychiatric consultation. It permits a careful and practical multidimensional assessment of the patient, his or her family and the treatment team and will facilitate interventions that will allow the consultant to collaborative with all parties, with the best interests of the patient in mind. In the table, we have used *italics* text to indicate relevant changes (e.g., pre-diagnosis and post-diagnosis), which may be the focus of clinical attention shifts in temperament are parallel shifts in the use of defense mechanisms (Chap. 2); Mr. Green begins to use of neurotic level defenses. Specifically, he employs denial to avoid consciously recognizing the severity of his cancer, suppression to compartmentalize his fear of the possible side effects or of death from the treatment, and he displaces his anxiety onto his family, becoming irritable and abrasive toward them. Finally, he approaches his family in a manner typical of a person who has a dismissive attachment style (Chap. 2), keeping his negative emotions private and preferring intellect over intimacy with his family. His family, unconsciously, and in a counter-phobic manner, makes the patient the scapegoat of the family-system crisis (Chap. 4).

Intervention by Psychiatric Consultant. In asking the patient's family members about Mr. Green's functioning and personality characteristics before the diagnosis, the consulting psychiatrist invites them to view Mr. Green in his former role as a strong family member who had maintained a stable system when others were in distress. Thereafter, the consultant focuses on helping Mr. Green consider, with the support of his family, a return to his previous stable level of functioning disrupted by his diagnosis and the recent deaths of his own parents. Using Table 3.2, the psychiatric consultant can quickly identify Mr. Green's strengths and initially "joins" and establishes an alliance with Mr. Green to encourage him recall his past in which he was admired by his family for his easy/ flexible temperament, humor, and the stabilizing role he had in their system.

The Family. Mr. Green's irritability makes it difficult for family members to be supportive. They feel pushed away and share with the psychiatric consultant that they have been accustomed to being cared for by Mr. Green when they are in distress, and consequently, they do not know how to be psychologically supportive to him.

Intervention by Psychiatric Consultant. Mr. Green's family is able to recognize that, though Mr. Green needs their support, they are coping with his personality changes by making him the scapegoat (Chap. 4). His wife and adult children are receptive to the consultant's recommendations and engage with Mr. Green, approaching him to talk about his fears, vulnerabilities, and need for support.

The Treatment Team. The members of the treatment team develop good rapport with the patient and his family and, recognizing their increased stress following the unexpected diagnosis of the testicular seminoma, suggest a psychiatric consultation. The recommendation is well received.

The Defiant Adolescent Patient Who Refuses Treatment

Jason, a 16-year-old who lives with his parents, is referred for a psychiatric consultation due to his refusal to continue with chemotherapy for Burkitt's lymphoma (Table 3.3).

Approximately a year and a half before his psychiatric consultation, Jason began to feel increasing fatigue and a general sense of malaise. After several

Table 3.3 Jason, the defiant adolescent patient who refuses treatment

	Patient before diagnosis	Patient after diagnosis	Family before diagnosis	Family after diagnosis	Treatment team members	Suggested consultant's intervention
Observed cognition	Flexible		Flexible		Flexible	• Given that both the patient and his family had flexible cognition, supportive psychodynamic intervention is appropriate
Observed temperament	Easy/flexible	*Slow to warm up*	Easy/flexible	Easy/flexible	Easy/flexible	• Focuses on the shift in the patient's observed temperament, defense mechanisms, attachment style
Observed defense mechanisms	Altruism Humor Sublimation	*Denial Suppression Displacement Intellectual-ization*				• "Joins" Jason and facilitates sharing the anger and frustration in having a serious illness • The consultant uses his alliance to help Jason share his ambivalence about continuing treatment
Observed attachment style	Secure	*Anxious*	Secure	Secure	Secure	• Supports the transition from observed relational patterns to his previously adaptive patterns
Family	Stable		Stable			• Engages Jason in discussing complex issues of adolescent independence and autonomy, which facilitated having the psychological space needed to make a decision to continue with his chemotherapy
Ethics		*Autonomy vs. beneficence*				

The table may be used to succinctly identify and assess the areas that require action by the psychiatric consultant in complex psychiatric consultation. It permits a careful and practical multidimensional assessment of the patient, his or her family, and the treatment team and will facilitate interventions that will allow the consultant to collaborate with all parties, with the best interests of the patient in mind. In the table, we have used *italics* to indicate relevant changes (e.g., pre-diagnosis and post-diagnosis), which may be the focus of clinical attention weeks of having these symptoms, he had a complete medical workup and was found to have Burkitt's lymphoma. Within a week, he was seen by a pediatric hematologist–oncologist and immediately began chemotherapy. His treatment was complicated by the development of tumor lysis syndrome when he only had five treatments remaining in his initial chemotherapy course. Jason refused to complete the last five treatments because of the side effects of the chemotherapy.

He stated to his family and to his hematologist–oncologist that he knew the risk of stopping chemotherapy. He shared that he was tired of suffering the intense nausea and vomiting after each of the treatments. He was also tired of having to suffer from the chemotherapy sequelae and feared dying due to his neutropenia. He no longer wanted to tolerate feeling terrible and preferred not to continue treatment.

His family became very concerned, and his hematologist–oncologist spoke with the family's pediatrician, who was close to them and was someone Jason trusted. The pediatrician was supportive and immediately suggested a psychiatric consultation to help understand Jason's motivation for wanting to stop treatment.

During the psychiatric consultation, Jason reported an unremarkable medical history up until the time of diagnosis. He conveyed a normal developmental history and an unremarkable family, educational, and social history. Thus, up until the discovery of the malignancy, Jason had a healthy and normal childhood and adolescence. The consulting psychiatrist learned from Jason's pediatrician and his hematologist–oncologist that Jason "handled most of his chemo treatments quite well and remained in relatively good spirits" in spite of the fact that his prognosis and response to the chemotherapy was uncertain. This information regarding the outcome was devastating to his parents, and though Jason was also affected by the uncertainty of his survival rate, his parents described him as "a really a strong kid" throughout the chemotherapy and said he handled the treatments well. Jason was a resilient adolescent, as demonstrated when as part of his treatment for his Burkitt's lymphoma he had to have portions of his eye orbit surgically removed and had to wear protective glasses, to prevent injuries when playing some sport activities. He had been an excellent tennis player, and though he could no longer play, he adjusted well to the restrictions brought about by his illness and seemed eager to continue living.

During the second meeting with the psychiatric consultant, without his parents present, Jason was cooperative and likable. He was very bright and had a good sense of humor despite the difficulties he was living through. He was not shy and promptly stated that he felt safe because his pediatrician had said that the consulting psychiatrist would be able to handle his feelings. Although he knew very little about the consultant, he seemed ready to share his feelings to anyone he felt would listen to him in a nonjudgmental way. He expressed frustration with the chemotherapy because he felt "terrible" afterward and also because—though he wanted to cry and yell—he felt he shouldn't because it would upset his mother. He said that he was not suicidal and added that he did not want to die. He pointed out that his hematologist–oncologist was unable to give any conclusive data about the potential for remission and, moreover, couldn't provide survival predictions that were different for 13 months versus 18 months of chemotherapy. Jason reasoned, "Science can't help me, so why should I continue?" He felt that the lack of conclusive data supported his stopping chemotherapy and was also angry at his hematologist–oncologist, who was acting like Jason was "a bad person for refusing treatment."

Jason recalled that on one occasion, his hematologist–oncologist and the oncology nurses had told him that he should be happy, because the side effects from the chemotherapy could not possibly be as bad as the effects of having untreated cancer. Clearly, Jason felt that there had been "an empathic failure" (Kohut 1966, Chap. 2) on the part of his oncology team, who could not see the chemotherapy from Jason's vantage. Jason wanted his side of the story to be heard, and he experienced the consulting psychiatrist as the external support he needed, knowing that the consultant would not be judgmental. Jason felt understood and readily agreed to be seen daily in the consultation process. He allowed the consulting psychiatrist to communicate with his pediatrician and the oncology team to help them grasp that Jason wanted to take "a short timeout" (a few days) to think carefully about his options rather than being pressured to make decisions. The psychiatric consultant—who had kept regular contact with the oncology treatment team—was cognizant that there was a very narrow window of time in which chemotherapy could be delayed and that, beyond this period, a delay could interfere with Jason's ability to complete the treatment regimen and to achieve a possible remission. Importantly, the consulting psychiatrist felt the typical countertransference reaction as a participating team member; that is, he noticed wanting to find a way to have Jason agree to continue with chemotherapy. Fortunately, the psychiatric consultant was able to allow himself to experience matters from Jason's vantage—from the inside out: "If science can't help him, why should he continue?"—very much like Stern's description of an intersubjective "present moment of meeting" (Stern 2004).

In subsequent meetings, Jason openly discussed his anger and sadness, which reflected his cognitive and affective flexibility and easy/flexible temperament style. Jason interacted well and shared some worries that indicated his positive outlook for his future. He wondered whether chemotherapy would affect his capacity to learn and to be successful later in his life. In fact, during one visit with the consulting psychiatrist, he asked if it would be okay for the two of them to go to the hospital cafeteria, so "we can talk about my cancer away from a 'medical room'." For the consulting psychiatrist, this "medical room" moment represented Jason's constant struggle and fear with medical procedures and hospitalizations. As the consultation continued, Jason gradually began to feel listened to and started wondering aloud if he should finish his remaining five chemotherapy treatments. He jokingly said that he did not know why, but "talking about this stuff helped me. I don't feel rushed or forced anymore." The following day Jason left a message at the psychiatric consultant's office, saying that he had agreed to finish his treatments and would call if he needed more help. In essence, the consultant had given Jason the space he needed to share his views on his dire situation and to carefully review his ambivalence about future chemotherapy treatments, while also providing him with time to manage the developmental and psychological struggles of adolescence (Delgado et al. 2012).

Jason's case illustrates the importance of listening to the patient and of actively participating in his experience. Often, we believe that careful and empathic listening can be helpful in itself, and while this is true, difficult psychiatric consultations like Jason's remind us that participating in our patient's struggles and in their ambivalence and dilemmas allows us to understand their experience. A system that creates a sense of mutuality between patient and the treatment team that cares for them communicates respect and often facilitates adherence to treatment recommendations.

Diagnostic Formulation and Interventions for Jason (Table 3.3). *The Patient.* Jason has a supportive family and a close relationship with his two older siblings, both of whom are high-achieving individuals. Thus, prior to the diagnosis of Burkitt's lymphoma, Jason functioned remarkably well from a psychological standpoint. He has excellent cognitive and affective flexibility, an easy/flexible temperament, a secure attachment style, mature defense mechanisms, and lives within a stable family system. The psychological changes after the diagnosis are expected and not reflective of psychopathology. Rather, these shifts represent individual and family crises. Jason is somewhat more anxious, fearful about his future, and begins to utilize more neurotic level defenses.

Intervention by Psychiatric Consultant. The consulting psychiatrist reassured Jason and helped to create the space needed for Jason to openly speak about his feelings and ambivalence regarding continuation of the chemotherapy treatment.

The Family. Jason's family was stable, supportive, and openly worked together, giving Jason the freedom to solve his dilemmas with the help of the psychiatric consultant.

Intervention by Psychiatric Consultant. The consultant provided support and empathically listened to the family's anxieties. This intervention was sufficient to permit the family to return to their pre-diagnosis relational patterns.

The Treatment Team. The members of the treatment team had developed good rapport with Jason, his parents, and his pediatrician, and recognized the difficulties on the part of the family and patient following the unexpected diagnosis of Burkitt's lymphoma. Thus, when the treatment team suggested a psychiatric consultation, it was welcomed by all.

Intervention by Psychiatric Consultant. The psychiatric consultant first established an alliance with the treatment team members, and later used his expertise to teach and model the ability to tolerate uncertainty regarding anticipated outcomes. In Jason's case, the treatment team's flexibility was of enormous help in allowing him to negotiate issues related to emerging adolescent autonomy in a healthy manner.

Ethics. This case illustrates difficult aspects of high-functioning adolescent patients' autonomy vs. nonmalfesience and also beneficence vs. nonmalfecense.

3.4   Summary

By inquiring into a patient's life story, with attention to his or her relationships with family, friends, and coworkers as well as to the person's accomplishments and hardships, the psychiatric consultant will glean invaluable information and will be able to better understand the patient's strengths and weakness. Such an understanding will almost certainly enhance treatment efforts and outcomes. Additionally, the reader should now appreciate that in approaching the *difficult psychiatric consultation*, it is critical to have a grasp of the patient's cognitive skills, capacity for cognitive and affective flexibility, and temperament styles. Systematically assessing the patient's defense mechanisms, personality and attachment styles, cognitive and affective flexibility, and temperament provide the psychiatric consultant with a window into why some of the members of a treatment team may have difficulty interacting with patient and his or her family and will inform the psychiatric consultant's interventions.

References

Altarac M, Saroha E (2007) Lifetime prevalence of learning disability among US children. Pediatrics 119:S77–S83

American Psychiatric Association (2013) Diagnostic and statistical manual of mental disorders, 5th edn. American Psychiatric Publishing, Washington, DC

Blackwell KA, Cepeda NJ, Munakata Y (2009) When simple things are meaningful: working memory strength predicts children's cognitive flexibility. J Exp Child Psychol 103:241–249

Bleiberg E (2000) Attachment, reflective function and the treatment of adolescents with severe personality disorder. In: Braconnier A, Gutton P (eds) Personality and conduct disorders in adolescents. GREUPP Paris, France, pp 365–381

Bowlby J (1999) Attachment: attachment and loss volume one, 2nd edn. Basic Books, New York, NY

Chess S, Thomas A, Birch HG et al (1960) Implications of a longitudinal study of child development for child psychiatry. Am J Psychiatry 117:434–441

Cooper S, Smiley E, Morrison J et al (2007) Mental ill-health in adults with intellectual disabilities: prevalence and associated factors. Br J Psychiatry 190:27–35

Delgado SV, Wassenaar E, Strawn JR (2011) Does your patient have a psychiatric illness or nonverbal learning disorder? Curr Psychiatr 10(5):17–35

Delgado SV, Strawn JR, Jain V (2012) Psychodynamic understandings. In: Levesque RJR (ed) Encyclopedia of adolescence. Springer, New York, NY, pp 2210–2219

Emde RN, Hewitt JK (2001) Infancy to early childhood: genetic and environmental influences on developmental change. Oxford University Press, Oxford

Frodl T, Skokauskasm N (2012) Meta-analysis of structural MRI studies in children and adults with attention deficit hyperactivity disorder indicates treatment effects. Acta Psychiatr Scand 125(2):114–126

Huizink A (2008) Prenatal stress exposure and temperament: a review. Eur J Dev Sci 2:77–99

Johnson DR (2009) Emotional attention set-shifting and its relationship to anxiety and emotion regulation. Emotion 9(5):681–690

Kagan J (1994) Galen's prophecy. Basic Books, New York, NY

Kagan J (2008) The biological contributions to temperaments and emotions. Eur J Dev Sci 2:38–51

Kohut H (1966) Forms and transformations of narcissism. J Am Psychoanal Assoc 14:243–272

Lai CH (2013) Gray matter volume in major depressive disorder: a meta-analysis of voxel-based morphometry studies. Psychiatry Res 211(1):37–46, Neuroimaging

Mahler S, Pine MM, Bergman A (1973) The psychological birth of the human infant. Basic Books, New York, NY

Mancia M (2006) Implicit memory and early unrepressed unconscious. Int J Psychoanal 87:83–103

McWilliams N (2011) Psychoanalytic diagnosis. Understanding personality structure in the clinical process, 2nd edn. Guilford Press, New York, NY, pp 21–42

Paulussen-Hoogeboom MC, Stams GJ, Hermanns JM et al (2007) Child negative emotionality and parenting from infancy to preschool: a meta-analytic review. Dev Psychol 43(2):438–453

Rothbart MK, Bates JE (2006) Temperament. In: Damon W, Lerner R (series eds), and Eisenberg N (volume ed) Social, emotional, and personality development, (6th ed.), vol 3. Handbook of child psychology. Wiley, New York, NY, pp 99–166

Schmeichel BJ, Volokhov RN, Demaree HA (2008) Working memory capacity and the self-regulation of emotional expression and experience. J Pers Soc Psychol 95(6):1526–1540

Schwartz CE, Wright CI, Shin LM et al (2003) Inhibited and uninhibited infants "grown up": adult amygdala response to novelty. Science 300:1952–1953

Steinberg L (2005) Cognitive and affective development in adolescence. Trends Cogn Sci 9 (2):69–74

Stern DN (2004) The present moment in psychotherapy and everyday life. WW Norton & Company, New York, NY, pp 135–149

Thomas A, Chess S (1977) Temperament and development. Brunner/Mazel, New York, NY

Thomas A, Chess S (1982) The reality of difficult temperament. Merrill Palmer Quart 28:1–20

Thomas A, Chess S (1986) The New York longitudinal study: from infancy to early adult life. In: Plomin R, Dunn J (eds) The study of temperament: changes, continuities, and challenges. Lawrence Erlbaum, Hillsdale, NJ

Thomas A, Chess S (1999) Goodness of fit: clinical applications from infancy through adult life. Routledge, New York, NY, pp 39–52

Thomas A, Chess S, Birch HG (1970) The origin of personality. Sci Am 223(2):102–109

Turner RJ, Roszell P (1994) Psychosocial resources and the stress process. In: Avison WR, Gotlib IH (eds) Stress and mental health: contemporary issues and prospects for the future. Plenum Press, New York, NY, pp 179–210

Webster RI, Erdos C, Evans K et al (2008) Neurological and magnetic resonance imaging findings in children with developmental language impairment. J Child Neurol 23(8):870–877

Zentner M, Bates JE (2008) Child temperament: an integrative review of concepts, research programs, and measures. Eur J Dev Sci 2(1/2):7–37

The Family

4

> *There is no doubt that it is around the family and the home*
> *that all the greatest virtues, the most dominating virtues of*
> *human society, are created, strengthened, and maintained*
> —Winston Churchill (1874–1965)

4.1 Dancing Together

The way that family members come to function as a unit can be likened to learning to dance. When families have learned to successfully dance with each other, there will be spoken and unspoken customs, rules, and patterns of behavior that are unique to them and yet serve the common goal of maintaining cohesion and stability of the family system. For some families, however, the dance reflects recurring patterns of conflict that provide a degree of cohesion but are still dysfunctional. In this chapter, we will describe a practical approach to common family systems conflicts and present some useful family-based and family-informed concepts that may be used in difficult psychiatric consultations. We will also review the importance that family systems theory has in consultation-liaison work. First, however, we will touch upon the early influence of family systems theory on psychiatry and child psychiatry.

4.2 Family Systems Theory

Family systems theory views families as being part of a dynamic and interactive system that changes over time. The main function of a family system is to support and nurture its members, and to promote their role as part of a larger collective community. The ways a particular family system supports and nurtures—that is, learns to dance with—each other develops over time according to the different temperaments, attachment styles, and personalities of each member. A family system is in essence the microcosm of a larger community and cultural system.

Winnicott (1966) stated that a baby cannot exist alone, but is essentially part of a relationship. Bowlby (1999) also recognized in his work that an infant cannot exist without a set of loving persons, preferably a larger family system that functions collaboratively to care for them. He further emphasized that a person's existence depends on the family system that has a past (before the person arrives) and a present (which includes the new member) and is part of a larger group, the community. The family system that functions well and is stable will intuitively know when a member needs support. It may be that a child with learning disabilities will require extra attention and time to complete their homework, or that an adult member with diabetes will need help following their diet.

It was during the early 1960s that general systems theory began to gain prominence in the scientific community, spearheaded by the work of the biologist Lvon (1950). He described systems as complex interactions between elements and used mathematical equations to indicate when systems were closed (if the elements did not have contact with the environment) and open (if they did). Family therapists excluded Bertalanffy's mathematical approach but took hold of the concept of open and closed systems. These systems seek "homeostasis," understood as the process by which a group of humans maintains a stable mode for survival. When the family system remains stable and balanced, then homeostasis is maintained and survival is assured. McConville and Delgado state that, earlier, "systemic approaches to family therapy were based on general systems theory, including the concept of cybernetics, which held that families tend to maintain equilibrium: a tension always exists between homeostasis and change, balancing stability and self-preservation with change and adaptation" (2006). The shift toward working with family systems had its origins in the social-work movement of the mid-1960s, when scholars and clinicians were dissatisfied with Freudian psychoanalytic theories. Ackerman, Minuchin, and Bowen—among the early family theorists who were analytically trained—found that general systems theory had many useful clinical applications to families and other social systems, and a number of distinct schools of family therapy began to emerge (Barker 1992; Hoffman 1981; Minuchin 1974; Minuchin and Fishman 1981). McConville and Delgado (2006) point out that "strategic and structural family therapies arose from this theory and focused on the observable as well as the reported family behavior" which is to say that several models of family therapy with different theoretical bases were developed, and though they had different theoretical bases, they shared an understanding of a family system's problem as evolving from the interplay of its members. Although a family may see a specific member as the "identified patient," the family therapist understands the problem as resting within the larger relational context of the family system as a whole. Therefore, in family systems theory, the diagnosis as such was not a central focus but rather the many unstable observable patterns of interaction seen in a family system.

Recognizing "unstable observable patterns of interaction" among family members is important during difficult psychiatric consultations. Not surprisingly, the work with families in such consultations can be quite challenging. It is essential to be familiar with family systems theory principles in order to address these issues and improve the outcome of the patient's treatment. When working with families of patients in difficult psychiatric consultations, the clinician should identify the strengths and weaknesses that existed in the family system before the diagnosis. Taking the time to understand the stable state a family may have had prior to the medical or psychiatric condition is extremely valuable in identifying how to best intervene and guide the family toward reestablishing their state of relative equilibrium. In reviewing with the patient and family their behaviors, rules, and styles of communication, the consultant can use this information to outline interventions that are respectful of the family's beliefs and customs. There will be significant changes in how a family system functions when coping with the inherent complexities of a medically or psychiatrically ill family member, and as such there will inevitably will be a recognizable "before and after the diagnosis" schism. In general, the psychiatric consultant's role is to help the treatment team provide resources that help the patient and family move as close as possible toward a known equilibrium to promote a shared common goal: the best outcome for the patient.

When the treatment team, patient, and family are engaged in conflict, the psychiatric consultant should keep in mind that the conflicts are multilayered and are influenced by the different expectations all parties have of each other. Helping these parties involves readjusting their energies to work toward a shared purpose— that of delivering the best care for the patient. When a patient has a serious medical or psychiatric illness, their known healthy historical self is set off balance, and consequently the family's stable historical collective self is also set off balance, as they are unable to tolerate the feelings of uncertainty and unpredictability the illness elicits in all. Once a stable system experiences the significant effects of the loss of predictability, it will promptly seek to regain it. How this change in the family system is displayed in the hospital or academic setting will be influenced by the interplay of all the family members' adaptive roles.

In designing interventions based his or her understanding of family systems concepts as well as his or her knowledge of the particular family involved, the psychiatric consultant helps the family "readjust" their priorities to allow for mature decisions with a minimal amount of conflict and to support their medically ill loved one.

When viewed through the family systems lens, the complicating factors that arise due to a patient's medical or psychiatric illness will move naturally, though perhaps with initial difficulty, toward homeostasis. Though subspecialty treatment teams are accustomed to treating people with illnesses that are similar, the patients' families all present with different configurations of bio-psycho-social complexities, which necessarily influence the outcome. There is no one solution to any set of family problems. The psychiatric consultant's role will be to explain to patient, family, and treatment team the impact that the medical or psychiatric condition has had on the emotional, relational, and cognitive strengths previously present. In more general terms, the usual family dance that existed before has now shifted. By understanding the patterns and identifying the patient's and family's unique needs, the psychiatric consultant can help treatment teams tailor their approach when delivering treatment plans, providing the patient and family with more informed expectations and a renewed level of encouragement.

Being diagnosed with a serious medical or psychiatric illness is frightening. When the condition is acute and known to respond to treatment, the family, although anxious, can reassure each other if there is a positive sense of predictability and certainty about the outcome. For example, knowing that the symptoms and changes in behavior of their loved one are the consequence of a viral upper respiratory tract infection is reassuring to the family, who understand that the condition will be short lived and that there is a high probability of a recovery. Furthermore, there is a sense of predictability and certainty about the treatment intervention, in this case with fluids and analgesics. The course and outcome are known factors, and balance is maintained. When the medical or psychiatric condition is acute but the course of treatment is unknown and complex, the homeostasis of the family is threatened, and issues of uncertainty and unpredictability arise. The reaction of a family system when one of its members is diagnosed with a serious medical or psychiatric illness is influenced by the unique and personal characteristics of each individual within the system. The reaction is further affected by the patient's personality style and ability to empathize of the medical providers who have completed the medical or psychiatric work-up, and the setting in which the diagnosis is delivered. When the diagnosis is delivered in the emergency room or on the medical unit, for instance, the loss of the family homeostasis is palpable. The response by the family members is also dependent on whether the quality of life of their loved one is likely to change.

Uncertainty and unpredictability are, of course, states that most would prefer not to experience. They may easily reawaken regressive patterns of behavior commonly used when under duress. The psychological threat created by the diagnosis of a serious illness can interfere with the welfare and cohesion of the family system. With the loss of homeostasis comes a new set of dilemmas about how this crisis should be handled among its members. The illness will elicit a completely different way of organizing relationships within the context of the family, with likely new polarities. Some families are resilient and adapt to change quite well, while others hang on to unrealistic wishes, struggling to accept that there has been a significant threat to their system. They may deny that their spouse, child, parent, or sibling is seriously ill and psychologically believe that soon everything will be "just fine, the way it was before."

Family Systems Theory in Difficult Consultations

The psychiatric consultant's goal in working with families should be to provide concise and practical recommendations to all members that can improve their role in supporting their loved one during the many difficult aspects of their illness. These recommendations should be determined according to what can be expected of the family system, which is intrinsically related to their collective functioning. If a treatment team is unable to help the patient and families manage feelings of anxiety and distress in the treatment planning meetings, the patient and family will be less able to participate in the decision-making process necessary for the implementation and delivery of optimal care. The psychiatric consultant can help by suggesting the treatment team assign one of its members to address the family's anxieties and explaining complex medical information. We have seen many cases in which the lead team member wants to "outsource" reassuring the family to a psychiatric consultant, believing it will take too much of his/her time. Despite this, the consultant with experience in family systems will facilitate the "dance" between patient, family, and team members, imbuing them with a sense of collective purpose. Of course, the consultant has limitations; he or she cannot make an angry and despondent family with temperamentally difficult/feisty members and with a disorganized attachment style become an easy/flexible family with a secure attachment style. Nevertheless, with the use of family systems concepts described later in this chapter, the consultant can help an angry family with a history of a disorganized attachment style learn to give priority to helping their family member, the patient, by allowing the treatment team to deliver and monitor the best-practice treatment needed, instead of engaging them in conflicted and unproductive interactions.

At the center of many requests for psychiatric consultation are family stressors not frequently recognized by the treatment team. When these stressors are not addressed early and with sensitivity, they can escalate rather quickly and lead to conflicts between family and treatment-team members. We have found that the most common family stressors, which are experienced as overwhelming, typically resolve after sensible interventions that can be implemented by the treatment teams (Josephson 2008). Unfortunately, families that are feeling overwhelmed do not often share their distress with treatment team, either from a sense of shame or the fear that they will receive lesser care if seen as "difficult." Among the common unrecognized family stressors are: (1) when the distance from home to the treatment facility is significant; (2) when the family has a history of prior losses due to complications from medical conditions; (3) when there is financial concern about the treatment needed (medications, follow-up visits, hospitalization). We suggest that the psychiatric consultant ask several simple questions to help identify the conflict triggers between the family and treatment team. The responses will guide the psychiatric consultant in formulating practical interventions that allow the parties involved to create a partnership with an agreement that their end goal is to provide the patient the best evidence-based treatment possible (Table 4.1).

We have seen difficult situations in which a family system is so distraught about caring for their loved one; they attempt to avoid participating in his or her care. When this happens, the treatment team may lose sight of the fact that there may be many psychological reasons that are overwhelming and affecting one or more of the family members expected to care for the patient. Upon observing that the family is not being attentive to their loved one, or not following the treatment recommendations, the team members may feel upset, perceiving that the family is either failing the patient or doesn't have his or her best interest in mind. To avoid this situation, the psychiatric consultant should encourage the team to learn about

Table 4.1 Questions about family stressors

• Is the distance from the patient's home to the treatment facility significant?

• Is there a history of losses in the immediate or extended family due to medical conditions?

• Do any members of the family have negative attitudes toward the medical field? If so, why?

• Do financial difficulties have a role in the family's daily life?

If so, financially, what aspects will be most affected by the hospitalization?

family members' ability to participate in their loved one's care. Currently, there is scant reference to assessing how the family system can participate within the context of a seriously ill child. There is still less attention given to the evaluation of the spouse, significant other, or family of adult patients. What references exist are found in literature regarding organ transplants, which emphasize the need to routinely perform a psychiatric-psychological evaluation of the patient prior to surgery "to help determine the capacity to consent, the presence of psychiatric disorders, the suicidality, and the potential for self-care" (Mamah et al. 2004). In addressing the case of children who need organ transplants, the importance is placed on the evaluation of parents (Afifi et al. 2006; Guadagnoli et al. 1999). We hope to see more research about the role family members have in the length of time needed for recovery when a member is diagnosed with a chronic serious illness. We recognize the importance of family systems and suggest that more attention be given to how family members, including siblings, function as a unit.

4.3   Family Systems Concepts

As in Chap. 2, in which we cherry-picked psychodynamic concepts relevant to consultation-liaison work, we have selected what we consider useful and practical concepts about family systems theory in understanding families. The following are terms commonly used in family systems theory to describe the dynamics when a stable state (homeostasis) is lost and conflict among members ensues, as often occurs in complex consultations (Table 4.2): joining, reframing, triangulation, scapegoating, generational boundaries, permeable boundaries, and family mapping or genogram.

Joining

This term is used to describe the rapport-building process necessary to allow the family therapist to make comments that facilitate communication among the family members with the therapist. Several rapport-building techniques that a therapist might use are: taking a one-down position (i.e., the consultant avoids the role of "expert" and empowers patient/family) without challenging the family's views, particularly when members have problems with authority figures; identifying common experiences, such as sports, cultural, or social events; matching the

Table 4.2 Common terms from family systems theory

• Joining: technique used to build rapport with family
• Reframing: giving new meaning to a behavior or set of interactions
• Triangulation: two family members, in conflict, attempt to enlist the support of a third ally
• Scapegoating: family projects problems on a particular member of their system
• Generational Boundaries: a family's age-related hierarchy on how to psychologically relate to each other
• Permeable Boundaries: boundaries susceptible to change due to patterns of closeness between family members
Family Mapping/Genogram: a visual display of a person's family tree

vocabulary used by the family. In difficult psychiatric consultations, joining with patient and family is essential for the consultant to be seen as someone who can broker the impasse that exists with the treatment team.

Reframing

"Reframing" refers to therapeutic approach in which the psychiatric consultant relabels the interactions between family members, providing a different perspective that increases awareness about the fact that a situation can have several "truths." This broadening of perspective gives the provider the space needed to change a negative pattern of interaction for a new one without feeling a loss of control over decisions.

The Pediatric Patient and Family Who Frustrate the Treatment Team

Melissa, an 11-year-old girl, is transferred from a community hospital to a large academic medical center after being diagnosed with an autoimmune encephalopathy. At the community hospital, in the context of her encephalopathy, Melissa's right arm was initially flailing uncontrollably, and she was yelling out words and was tremulous. Moreover, she appeared to be responding to internal stimuli and actively experiencing visual hallucinations. Upon her arrival at the academic medical center, her care is assumed by the neurology service, and plasmapheresis is initiated to treat her encephalopathy. A parenteral antipsychotic, olanzapine, is begun to treat the patient's delirium, but over 2 days, the neurologists find that olanzapine only minimally improves her delirium. At that time, a psychiatric consultation is requested.

Initially, the attending neurologist had informed Melissa's parents, with empathy and honesty, that their daughter's autoimmune encephalopathy could be fatal or might leave her with a chronic mental disability that would prevent her return to a functional state. Melissa's parents began to cry and said that they wanted their daughter to be medicated to keep her from "knocking things over and screaming out." The neurologist agreed, though also expressed that it was best not to overmedicate Melissa because they would not be able to assess

Table 4.3 The pediatric patient and family who frustrate the treatment team

	Patient before diagnosis	Patient after diagnosis	Family before diagnosis	Family after diagnosis	Treatment team members	Suggested consultant's intervention
Observed cognition	Good	Impaired	Good	*Limited/ good*	*Inflexible*	• Helps the treatment team members recognize their own fear in having to deliver potentially devastating news to caring, although overwhelmed parents has led them to take a rather inflexible approach to the case. • Reminds the treatment team of parents strengths, prior to daughter's illness.
Observed temperament	Easy/ flexible	Difficult/feisty	Easy/ flexible	*Difficult/ feisty*	*Slow to warm up*	• Facilitates parents, and treatment team members, recognition of common goals and the need to develop a collaborative partnership.
Observed defense mechanisms	Mature	Self-injurious behaviors	Mature	*Immature*	*Neurotic*	• Encourages the treatment team to provide ample time for questions when explaining to parents the seriousness of daughter's condition. • Shares and discusses experience in other similar cases to reassure parents of their approach to the condition.
Observed attachment style	Secure	Insecure	Secure	*Anxious*	*Anxious*	• Helps parents discuss fears. • Provides the psychological space for the patient's parents to feel safe and to share their frustrations with the treatment team and gradually help them reflect that some of their frustrations relate to their own fear of vulnerability.
Family	Scapegoat		Stabilizer (under crisis)	*Scapegoat*		• Helps parents identify factors that led them to retreat from their typical stabilizing roles.

The table may be used to succinctly identify and assess the areas that require action by the psychiatric consultant in complex psychiatric consultation. It permits a careful and practical multidimensional assessment of the patient, his or her family, and the treatment team and will facilitate interventions that will allow the consultant to collaborate with all parties, with the best interests of the patient in mind. In the table, we have used *italics* to indicate relevant changes (e.g., pre-diagnosis and post-diagnosis), which may be the focus of clinical attention whether her mental status and neurologic condition were improving or worsening.

During the same conversation the neurologist shared with the parents a desire to involve social services, who would make arrangements for them to temporarily stay at a local hospital-affiliated facility where they could have some reprieve from the hospital, would be able to change clothes, shower, etc. Melissa's parents became irritated and told the team, "No, we don't need a social worker," and thereafter refused to speak with any of the neurology team members. Fortunately, they felt understood by the nursing staff, which relayed their questions, observations, and requests to the neurology team.

The psychiatric consultant reviewed the information available, met with neurology team, and met with Melissa's parents (Table 4.3). The consultation-liaison team, after introducing their members—attending psychiatrist, resident, and fellow—and explaining why the neurologist had requested the consult, shared with Melissa's parents that they believed quetiapine could be helpful in managing their daughter's agitation (Turkel et al. 2012). Shortly after this discussion, the parents had a "meltdown" in the intensive care unit where Melissa was receiving plasmapheresis, and they "cussed out" the neurology team, blaming their daughter's agitation on the new medication, although the behavioral chart indicated it had actually lessened. At that point, the neurology team became frustrated with the psychiatric consultants, saying, "You need to tell the parents that they cannot behave like this," adding, "If they are not going to allow us to treat their daughter how we think is best, we might have to transfer her to another hospital." The psychiatric consultant, in an effort to use this as a teachable moment, spoke with the neurology team about the difficulty that Melissa's parents had had: they were being asked to cooperate with complete strangers when in fact their daughter could die at any minute. The key member of the neurology team replied, "Well, the parents are really going through a lot, and they must be angry that are going to lose their healthy daughter. They actually are doing their best. I will go later and speak with them about all of the options and the importance treating her delirium appropriately."

Later that day, the consulting psychiatrist spoke with Melissa's parents at length and observed, "It seems there's something about using this particular medication that really frightens you." They replied that Melissa's mother had worked in a nursing home and felt that the nursing home staff "would just keep the patients sedated all day long with that antipsychotic, and they looked like zombies." The consultant was able to join with Melissa's parents in feeling powerless and reframed the need for the medication as something that would help the patient with her discomfort and agitation, rather than sedate her. Also, the consultant used a "one-down position" in which he asked Melissa's parents, "Would you consider allowing us to use quetiapine, just a few more doses, to help with Melissa's agitation?"

Using a family systems approach, joining, the consulting team asked Melissa's parents what their daughter's summer had been like and how had she'd done at school before the illness. In tears, Melissa's parents told the team that the summer had been fun, adding that Melissa enjoyed swimming, that she was a "straight A student," and had been eagerly looking forward to sixth grade. They had clearly begun the mourning process of their high-achieving daughter and were struggling with the feeling any psychologically healthy parent would have, not wanting to accept such a sad reality.

Diagnostic Formulation and Interventions for Melissa (Table 4.3). *The Patient.* Melissa exhibits psychological and cognitive changes consistent with her autoimmune encephalopathy, which requires pharmacological interventions to address secondary agitation. In this case, the shift in observed temperament, defense mechanisms, and attachment style after being diagnosed with autoimmune encephalopathy are clearly not amenable to psychological intervention by the consulting psychiatry team.

Intervention by Psychiatric Consultant. The psychiatry team makes pharmacological recommendations to decrease the patient's agitation.

The Family. Melissa's parents manage their anxieties, fears, and anger about their daughter's serious condition by projecting onto the treatment-team members, and they perceive the treatment team as not being supportive, believing members act in a negative way toward their daughter: "They just want to medicate her so she can be like a zombie." The healthy and stable system that allowed Melissa to be a high-achieving adolescent prior to her illness was abruptly disrupted by the autoimmune encephalopathy. The acute onset of the illness led the usually high-functioning parents to suddenly transition to observed difficult/feisty temperaments, limitations in cognitive and affective flexibility, and the use of immature defense mechanisms.

Intervention by Psychiatric Consultant. In using this Table 4.3, the consulting team identifies Melissa's parents' strengths and provides the psychological space they need to feel safe and share the frustration they've experienced with the treatment-team members. The psychiatry team also gradually helps them reflect on the fact that perhaps some of their frustrations represent their own fear of vulnerability and the need to mourn their formerly high-achieving adolescent. This allows them to collaborate with the treatment team in the difficult decision-making process that lies ahead due the severity of their daughter's condition.

The consulting team uses their alliance to encourage the parents to allow themselves to be helped as they grapple with being in the new territory of having a daughter suffering from autoimmune encephalopathy. Her parents are guided in learning that in order to help their daughter, it is necessary to collaborate with the treatment team, and to do so they need to return to their former stabilizing role in the family system.

The Treatment Team. The members of the treatment team begin by asking Melissa's parents to agree with urgent decisions about the psychopharmacologic intervention needed for their daughter's agitation without first establishing rapport with them. Melissa's neurologist transforms from a high-functioning provider to a provider with significant countertransference reactions and shifts to a slow-to-warm-up temperament style, uncharacteristic cognitive and affective inflexibility, and the use of neurotic defense mechanisms.

Intervention by Psychiatric Consultant. In using this table, the consulting team identifies that the treatment team needs to establish rapport with the patient's parents and help them realize that the family system, up to Melissa's admission for the autoimmune encephalopathy, was functioning with remarkable stability. The psychiatry team, in discussing the case with the treatment team, raises the possibility that their own fear of explaining the seriousness of the patient's condition to her parents does not allow the family to ask questions.

Triangulation

This is a process commonly seen when family members who are in conflict with each other seek to involve a third person (e.g., parent, child, therapist), with the hope of deflecting intensity away from themselves. For example, in a married couple, the father tells his son about the dissatisfaction he has with the child's mother—his wife—for not helping the child with his homework and adds that the mother is responsible for the child's poor grades. The mother, on other occasions, tells the child that it is his father's—her husband's—negativity that causes both of them to experience depression, which is why she cannot help her son with his homework, and his poor grades are his father's fault. Thus, their son is used as the third person by both parents in their triangulation.

In the clinical setting this may occur when a family member demands that the psychiatric consultant agree with their view on how to proceed with the medical or psychiatric treatment, against the wishes of the patient, who has agreed with the initial recommendations of the treatment team. The intent of the family member may be to triangulate with the psychiatric consultant and avoid repeating the long-term conflicts that have existed among the family members and the patient, who is now viewed as being allied with the treatment-team members. Although this scenario is detrimental to the best-care treatment plan for the patient, it is helpful in revealing the underlying tensions that exist between the patient and their family. The psychiatric consultant will need to help the family find common ground with the patient and minimize the need to triangulate. The concept of triangulation can also be useful when working in difficult psychiatric consultations, as it can be employed with sensitivity in a therapeutic manner. For example, the psychiatric consultant may choose to temporarily ally with the family member in distress to reduce their anxiety and to jointly review the pros and cons of the complicated decisions regarding the patient's treatment plan. Though the treatment team may initially feel confused as to why the psychiatric consultant is aligning with the family, in time they recognize that in doing so the psychiatric consultant diffused the family conflict, and, by joining with the family member, improved their stance about supporting the treatment team's plan for the patient.

The Adult Patient Who Triangulates with the Help of His Wife

A 42-year-old man is admitted for the treatment of his depression after attempting to overdose with his antidepressants while his wife was on vacation. The patient requests that his wife not share with the treatment team that he had not been taking the antidepressant as prescribed or keeping his psychotherapy appointments. He promises his wife that it will not happen again, in spite of the fact that over the last several months this has been his pattern—not following through with his treatment. Sadly, the patient's wife agrees to this triangulation as she is in a bind. If she shares the information with the treatment team, her husband will be upset and mistrust her, although she also recognizes that withholding the information will interfere with the treatment team's decisions and that they may discharge her husband without careful review of a safety plan. This example bears out that it is imperative for treatment teams to routinely seek collateral information from as many parties as possible, especially after a patient attempts to end his or her life. In this case, the psychiatric consultant's communication with the patient's psychiatrist and psychotherapist brought to light the problem of noncompliance, and an in-depth family intervention is recommended. The consultant uses this information to join with the patient and reframe that his wish for secretiveness (triangulating with his wife to hide important information from the treatment team) will likely lead to further failure. This intervention also helps his wife, as she no longer feels compelled to withhold valuable information to ensure her husband's trust. She has been loyal to his request. The patient could use this opportunity to speak to his wife about his anger over her vacation, which made him feel "left alone to cope with my depression." This of course is a clear instance where marital therapy will be recommended upon discharge. The psychiatric consultant, pointing out to the patient his counterproductive strategy and encouraging him to confide in the treatment team about his difficulties with compliance and self-defeating behavior, allows for the development of practical aftercare plans (Table 4.4).

Diagnostic Formulation and Interventions for the Depressed Patient (Table 4.4). *The Patient.* There are clear changes in the patient's observed temperament, his increased use of neurotic defense mechanisms, and the triangulation with his wife to prevent the treatment team from learning about his self-defeating behaviors. Where his temperament has been characteristically easy/flexible, after his overdose attempt, we see a shift to a difficult/feisty temperament, and he begins to deny the severity of the depression. Outwardly his interactions with others are similar to those of an individual with a dismissive attachment style.

Intervention by Psychiatric Consultant. It becomes apparent that interventions should focus on the patient's self-defeating behaviors and facilitate his return to his state of psychological health disrupted by his increased symptoms of depression and hopelessness. In using this (Table 4.4), the consultant identifies the patient's strengths and first "joins" with him, encouraging him

Table 4.4 A 42-old man is admitted for the treatment of major depressive disorder

	Patient before diagnosis	Patient after diagnosis	Family before diagnosis	Family after diagnosis	Treatment team members	Suggested consultant's intervention
Observed cognition	Inflexible		Inflexible		Flexible	• Given that both the patient and his wife are cognitively rigid, problem-oriented psychoeducational and supportive interventions are needed.
Observed temperament	Easy/flexible	Difficult/feisty	Slow to warm up	Slow to warm up	Easy/flexible	• After noting that the temperament of the patient has changed and that his wife's temperament remains stable, the consultant focuses on the shift in the patient's observed temperament, defense mechanisms, attachment style, and on his role within his marriage. The consultant joins the patient and "reframes" his wish for secretiveness to facilitate sharing of his feelings of shame and guilt about his illness, and in doing so the consultant facilitates increased support from the patient's wife and treatment team.
Observed defense mechanisms	Altruism Intellectualization Sublimation	*Denial Suppression Displacement*		*Denial Suppression Displacement*		
Observed attachment style	Secure	*Dismissive*	Secure	*Anxious*	Secure	
Family	Stabilizer	*Scapegoat*		*Triangulation between patient and wife*		• Joins and reframes with the patient that his wish for secretiveness will lead to further failure and that it is a counterproductive strategy and encourages him to confide in his wife and treatment team about his difficulties with compliance. • Helps the patient engage his wife in order to prevent future triangulations by asking for her support to help him manage his medications and outpatient appointments and improve compliance for further success.

The table may be used to succinctly identify and assess the areas that require action by the psychiatric consultant in complex psychiatric consultation. It permits a careful and practical multidimensional assessment of the patient, his or her family, and the treatment team and will facilitate interventions that will allow the consultant to collaborate with all parties, with the best interests of the patient in mind. In the table, we have used *italics* text to indicate relevant changes (e.g., pre-diagnosis and post-diagnosis), which may be the focus of clinical attention to share his frustrations. The consultant follows by "reframing" the patient's wish for secretiveness as a counterproductive strategy. The patient is encouraged to confide in the treatment team about his difficulties with compliance. Additionally, given the patient's relatively rigid cognitive style, the consultant provides education regarding the chronicity of depressive disorders, which may require further hospitalizations.

The Family. The patient's wife is put in a difficult position by her husband's unrealistic wishes for secrecy, and this accentuates her fears for his safety.

Intervention by Psychiatric Consultant. The psychiatric consultant helps the patient to allow his wife to become a partner in the treatment of his depression. Her loyalty and active support will aid in preventing setbacks and create a better outlook for their future.

The Treatment Team. The members of the treatment team have good rapport with the patient and family and, recognizing their stress in coping with depression, suggest a psychiatric consultation.

Intervention by Psychiatric Consultant. The psychiatric consultant removes the treatment team from possible triangulation between the patient and his wife, helping the patient understand that his wish for secretiveness is a counterproductive strategy and encouraging him to confide in his wife and treatment team about his difficulties with compliance. The consultant also encourages the treatment team to explain to the patient and wife that setbacks during the course major depressive disorder are not uncommon.

Scapegoating

"Scapegoating" is similar to triangulation, although it describes the attempt to resolve the conflict between two or more family members by displacing the conflict onto a different family member. The person recruited, albeit unconsciously, to serve as the scapegoat is usually the patient. Often in hospitals or academic settings, though treatment team may view the family as interfering with the patient's progress by not supporting the medical or pharmacological recommendations, the family members themselves do not consider their behavior unreasonable. Rather they claim that it is their medically or mentally ill member who is being unreasonable for refusing to take his or her medication, in spite of the fact that the patient has been coached by the family to refuse treatment. The family's anxiety in collaborating with the treatment team is diffused by using the patient as a scapegoat: "He is the one being difficult, not us." This is common for families whose past experiences with others have been characterized as passive/aggressive due to their temperament and attachment vulnerabilities. Although they consciously fear conflict, they unknowingly create it.

Using the Child as a Scapegoat

The mother of a 12-year-old boy with poorly-controlled asthma and frequent asthma attacks systematically singles him out when things go wrong at home. He is blamed for "keeping the family stressed" due to his asthma because "We can't do anything without you getting sick." His mother expresses her anger about his hospitalizations as she is required to attend bedside treatment-team rounds and family meetings, which she experiences as inconvenient and taking time away from her other children. The psychiatric consultant, with help from the treatment team, joins with the mother and reframes the problem by explaining that it is not the child who keeps the family stressed, it is his illness—asthma—that stresses the family system, including the child. This helps his mother appreciate that the child is not to blame and providing education about his asthma may reduce the family stress. Needless to say, this family will not change overnight simply because the consultant has helped the mother differentiate her son from his asthma. Due to the chronicity of their family difficulties, a case manager refers them to home healthcare services, which can hopefully ensure the adherence to his medication and help the family system change over time.

Generational Boundaries

These are invisible lines of separation between generations within the context of the family system and its cultural background. In the Hispanic culture it is common for the adult child to live at home while attending college or working toward a postgraduate degree, while in USA it is more common for the young adult to live away from home during this time and maintains regular contact with daily or weekly calls to parents. In both situations, healthy generational boundaries encourage parents to maintain culturally relevant parental roles and their children to maintain developmentally appropriate roles.

As an example: A couple composed of an American mother and a Hispanic father has their first child, a girl. Soon after birth, the father's mother requests that her granddaughter have her ears pierced while in the nursery, as is customary in Mexican culture, with the gold earrings she has specially bought. The pediatrician, whom the parents trust, informs the parents of the benefit in waiting to have her ears pierced until their child is older, as is customary in the USA. The child's father is able to openly discuss the pressures of the generational boundary with his mother, and although they are initially conflicted, they find a compromise through a Hispanic baptism, delaying the child's ear piercing.

The issue of generational boundaries can become complicated in difficult psychiatric consultations, and the consultant will benefit from paying attention to its spoken and unspoken manifestations within the family systems. In some situations, when the parents of adult patients with serious medical or psychiatric illnesses are overwhelmed by uncertainty and the unpredictability of the situation, they unconsciously wish to return to a time when they had an authoritative role in the life of their adult child, which may feel to the patient as undermining his or her autonomy. On the other hand, some adult patients will disagree with their parents in order to maintain a sense of independence, in spite of the fact that the parents have a more realistic view of the treatment plan. Still other patients may fear challenging the generational boundaries and allow the older parents to make the decisions even if these seem not to be made in a thoughtful and reasonable manner. The psychiatric consultant can help by joining with the family and reframing the situation in a way that allows for a productive discussion about the generational boundaries, whereby all members feel included in the outcome and continue with best-practice treatment recommendations.

Generational boundaries within the family system may play out in an unspoken manner in a variety of ways in the medical setting. For example, the age of treatment-team members may impact the patient's decision-making, especially when the physicians, residents, and other support staff are significantly younger than the patient and family. Because of the age difference, the family may fear of not being understood regarding their beliefs and family values, seeing the treatment team as "inexperienced and too young" and disagree with the treatment recommendations, requesting to be seen by a senior physician. This may also apply to the recently minted psychiatric consultant. In any case, such generational anxieties are best addressed in an open manner, with members of the treatment team first sharing the level of experience they have. Most families are happily surprised by the expertise of a young physician or psychiatric consultant. Second, it is important to ask what the family wishes to teach the consultant and treatment team about their own values, worries, and fears. We have found this empathic approach effective in most difficult psychiatric consultations, although not with families that have a history of difficult/feisty temperaments and insecure, disorganized attachment. In these situations, a seasoned clinician, or a consulting team, may be in a better position to help.

Permeable Boundaries

This describes a dynamic in which family members encourage the exchange of information among them. Such a dynamic can be helpful in the medical setting, when a family with mutually trusting relationships enables a mature sharing and discussion of medical information provided by treatment teams. The informed loved ones, upon sharing these details with family members who are not present, contribute to a state of cohesiveness and community. For example, when man with hypercholesterolemia has a myocardial infarction, his family can support him by making changes to its menus and limiting certain foods for all members in the home. In a well-adjusted family system, the permeability facilitates cooperation through a mutual agreement to share the diagnosis and treatment recommendations of an ill family member with others who later can provide support.

In unstable and dysfunctional family systems, the permeability of boundaries is usually detrimental in working with a patient. This process can be seen in families where one member develops an eating disorder, usually an adolescent. The patient's family has difficulty maintaining clear boundaries, and problems with permeable boundaries, known as family "enmeshment," occur. When this happens, the family collectively avoids confronting the self-defeating behaviors of their loved one. The patient is able to convince the family to ask for compassion from the treatment team and avoid aggressive interventions needed (e.g., nasal-gastric tube for feeding). The patient may also have family members collude with them in sabotaging the treatment by skipping meals without letting the team know. Typically, the parents or spouse challenge the treatment team's recommended interventions, insisting these make the patient feel worse and that they know more about what would help their family member.

The Adult Patient Who Sabotages Treatment

Mrs. Jones, a 30-year-old African American with a psychiatric history remarkable for major depressive disorder and a long physical history of poorly controlled type II diabetes, has an HbA_1C of 11 % (normal range: 4–6.4 %) and has been on an insulin regimen for 3 years prior to her hospitalization. During the course of an admission for diabetic hyperosmolar coma (a condition in which hyperglycemia produces extreme dehydration and increases in serum osmolality), her hospitalist and endocrinologist note that she has poor capacity to carefully manage her blood sugar, and in fact frequently sabotages her treatment by eating foods containing high-fructose corn syrup. At times, Mrs. Jones puts honey under her fingertips so as to artificially elevate her finger-stick blood sugar readings. Also, her hospitalist is frustrated by the fact that Mrs. Jones has had multiple prior admissions to the medical unit due to her mismanagement of her diabetes. The various hospitalists who have cared for Mrs. Jones in the past recognize her tendency to sabotage matters, and her current hospitalist requests a psychiatric consultation, the fourth in a 6-month period. Mrs. Jones's situation is further complicated in that she conspires with her mother, who frequently brings her food that clearly will affect her blood glucose. When told repeatedly by members of the nursing staff that Mrs. Jones cannot eat the homemade brownies she brings to the hospital, her mother becomes upset and angry and at times berates the nursing staff. On one such occasion, during an argument between Mrs. Jones' mother and the nursing staff, the attending endocrinologist urgently calls upon the psychiatric consultant to help the treatment team. The consultant recognizes that Mrs. Jones and her mother have projected onto the treatment team their own limited capacity to tolerate the sadness about the severity and chronicity of Mrs. Jones' diabetes and the implications of this on their lives. Telling the treatment team that he will intentionally be *joining* with the family's projections of them, agreeing that the team's recommendations seem punitive, the consultant explains that this intervention will allow him to *reframe* the problem. Discussing the conflict with the patient and her mother, the consultant states, "It's almost like they're saying you to give up everything that you enjoy—the sweets, the brownies, everything." At this point, he adds, "What if we talk to them [the treatment team] and ask them to educate us in terms of how many brownies it would be possible to eat if you both agree to follow their recommendations?" By including himself in the projected criticism of the treatment team, the consultant is able to embark on the process of limit-setting. Importantly, his intent is not to change the long-standing cognitive, temperament, and attachment styles but rather to "plant a seed" by temporarily allowing the family to align with the medical provider, an alliance that may be utilized in subsequent hospitalizations or consultations.

In approaching this case, the psychiatric consultant noted that the patient's family generally was dismissive of the treatment team's recommendations and frequently used denial. He also noticed the permeability of boundaries within the family system. To address these issues, the psychiatric consultant continued to join the patient and her mother's projections onto the treatment team, and because of this joining, he was able to more successfully establish limits that, over time, were better tolerated by the patient and her mother (Table 4.5).

Diagnostic Formulation and Interventions for Mrs. Jones (Table 4.5).
The Patient. It is helpful for the psychiatric consultant to know that Mrs. Jones' hospitalist and endocrinologist noted that she has poor capacity to carefully manage her blood glucose, and that in spite of several hospital admissions for her diabetes, she frequently sabotages her treatment by eating foods containing high-fructose corn syrup, confirming a history of limited and concrete cognitive abilities. Sadly, the patient and her mother display chronic vulnerabilities with persistent temperament difficulties, use of immature defense mechanisms, permeable boundaries, and with an insecure attachment style.

Intervention by Psychiatric Consultant. Noting that the patient's behavior is part of a chronic, self-defeating pattern of treatment sabotage, and that both the patient and her mother had minimal cognitive flexibility, the consulting psychiatrist recognizes the limitations of their ability to comply with treatment recommendations and helps the treatment team develop, in writing, concrete behavioral expectations, and educational interventions that can be referred to if further admissions occur.

The Family. The patient's mother shows signs of enmeshment behavior with permeable boundaries, frequently bringing her food that clearly will affect her blood glucose, knowing that her adult daughter is not participating actively in her treatment.

Intervention by Psychiatric Consultant. The consultant joins with the patient and mother, with sensitivity, understanding that they have been experiencing the treatment recommendations as punitive. The consultant reframes the problem, allowing him to embark on the process of limit-setting. In this regard, the psychiatric consultant opened a discussion: "it's almost like they're saying that your daughter has to give up everything that you enjoy, the sweets, the brownies, everything." At this point, he added "What if we talk to them [the treatment team] and ask them to educate us in terms of how many brownies would be possible to eat if you both agree to follow their recommendations?" By including himself in the projected criticism of the team, he enables the patient and her

Table 4.5 The adult patient who sabotages treatment

	Patient before diagnosis	Patient after diagnosis	Family before diagnosis	Family after diagnosis	Treatment team members	Suggested consultant's intervention
Observed cognition	Impaired	Impaired	Impaired	Impaired	Flexible	• Given that both the patient and her mother have limited cognition, the consultant helps the treatment team to develop concrete limit-setting and educational interventions needed.
Observed temperament	Difficult/feisty	Difficult/feisty	Difficult/feisty	Difficult/feisty	Easy/flexible	• After noting that the patient's and family's temperament, defense mechanisms, and attachment style have a long history of instability, the consultant suggests that the treatment team provide the patient decisions made about setting limits in written form—visitation time, food and off unit restrictions, etc.—and initiate a process of collaborative work with social services to assure home health care after discharge.
Observed defense mechanisms	Immature	Immature	Immature	Immature	Mature	
Observed attachment style	Insecure/dismissive	Insecure/dismissive	Insecure/dismissive	Insecure/dismissive	Secure	• Helps the patient and her mother recognize that their self-defeating behaviors necessitated inpatient psychiatric treatment.
Role in family	Scapegoat	Scapegoat	Permeable boundaries Enmeshment			
Ethics	Autonomy vs. beneficence Impaired capacity					• Evaluates patient's medical decision making capacity.

The table may be used to succinctly identify and assess the areas that require action by the psychiatric consultant in complex psychiatric consultation. It permits a careful and practical multidimensional assessment of the patient, his or her family and the treatment team and will facilitate interventions that will allow the consultant to collaborate with all parties, with the best interests of the patient in mind. In the table, we have used *italics* to indicate relevant changes (e.g., pre-diagnosis and post-diagnosis), which may be the focus of clinical attention mother to accept recommendations in a less combative manner. He also establishes an alliance that may be used later in consultation or treatment.

The Treatment Team. The members of the treatment team were frustrated with the patient's self-defeating behavior and had begun to act out their countertransference feelings, saying, "They are borderline. We can't do anything else for them." Thus, in parallel processes, the team members were distancing themselves from the patient and mother, just as the patient and mother were distancing themselves from the team.

Intervention by Psychiatric Consultant. The psychiatric consultant helps the treatment team recognize their countertransference feelings and aids their reengagement by providing, in writing, decisions made about behavioral expectations—visitation time, food, and off-unit restrictions, etc. If appropriate, the consultant may share the papers by Groves (1978) and Strous et al. (2006), reviewed in Chap. 2, to provide teachable moments on self-defeating patients. Initiating a process of collaborative work with social services, the consultant assures home health care after discharge.

Ethics. This case raises issues about the need to evaluate the patient in terms of the patient's capacity to give or withhold consent.

Intervention by Psychiatric Consultant. The consultant recommends more intensive (inpatient) psychiatric treatment in order to gain a better understanding of the patient's strength and weakness. It is particularly important to tease out whether the patient's self-defeating behaviors are secondary to her cognitive limitations or related to a personality disorder that may be more responsive to an inpatient supportive and structured environment.

4.4   Genograms: Family Mapping

Genograms, which are also referred as *family mapping*, are visual diagrams of a family's organizational structure, alliances, and boundaries. In consultation-liaison psychiatry, the genogram does not have to be complete. Rather it can be limited to immediate and close family members, as long as it captures the most pertinent features of the family system. Helping the patient and family create a genogram can be quite useful in that it allows them to review and recognize their roles within the family system prior to the diagnosis of the medical or psychiatric illness. A genogram is also a useful visual tool for the treatment team, aiding their understanding of how the patient served the family system prior to illness. Using this tool, the psychiatric consultant may identify the family member best equipped emotionally to provide support for the patient, may discover the way certain psychiatric illnesses (e.g., depression and anxiety disorders) have manifested throughout the family, as well as the way these illness might have affected intergenerational relationships. It can also help identify the family members who may need the most attention and hand-holding (if they are close to and dependent on their ill loved one), as a means of avoiding unnecessary burden on the patient. Along this line, if the genogram reveals that the patient has been the source of conflict with certain family members, the consultant and treatment team can design a list of those allowed to visit, thus preventing family conflicts at the patient's bedside. The genogram can also pinpoint the family members with whom the patient wishes to share treatment information and may facilitate discussions of matters of confidentiality, end-of-life decisions, etc.

At times patients and their families are so overwhelmed by coping with the illness that has resulted in hospitalization; they find it a relief when the treatment or consulting team takes the lead in sharing information about the patient's condition. Upon reviewing the genogram, the team may find a sibling or relative whom the family described as "levelheaded and supportive" and may reach out to him or her.

How to Create a Genogram

Ideally, the genogram will show relationships diagrammatically, and several conventions are used in demarcating these relationships (Wachtel 1982; McGoldrick et al. 1999). Typically, squares are used to represent males and circles to represent females. X's indicate that an individual is deceased, and circles around individuals reflect that they live within a single household. Two diagonal lines crossing a "relationship line" signify divorce, while a single line denotes separation. Siblings are typically listed in birth order from right to left (Fig. 4.1). An example of genogram of a patient with idiopathic scoliosis is shown in Fig. 4.2. The psychiatric consultant was able to use the genogram to understand the relationship between the patient and his older sister, who—although away at college—had previously served in a mother role for the patient. The consultant also employed the diagram to explain to the treatment team the way in which the patient, who was the youngest child in a family of very high achieving individuals, regressed as the upcoming scoliosis surgery approached.

4.5 The Family in Child and Adolescent Psychiatry

Over the last two decades, there has been significant controversy over whether families of children and adolescents should take part in the decision-making processes of their psychiatric treatment. The main concern was that the families, because of their limited medical knowledge and reliance on unscientific information (often obtained from the internet), would be unwilling to follow the treatment team's best-practice medical recommendations. Needless to say, the fears about the family interfering with the treatment were unsubstantiated. Rather, when families contributed in the decision-making process with medical providers, the care and outcome of children and adolescents receiving treatment were improved. This early controversy led to the creation of a *Bill of Rights* (AACAP 2008), which was adopted by the mental health declaration of human rights, in which mentally ill

Fig. 4.1 Approach to
constructing a family
genogram

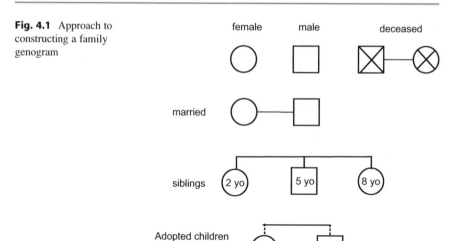

patients and their families are encouraged to have a shared role in the implementation of the treatment plan. In 2008, the children's mental health coalition created a *Bill of Rights for Children with Mental Health Disorders and their Families*. The coalition included members from the American Academy of Child and Adolescent Psychiatry (AACAP), Children and Adults with Attention-Deficit/Hyperactivity Disorder (CHADD), the Autism Society of America (ASA), the Child and Adolescent Bipolar Foundation (CABF), the Federation of Families for Children's Mental Health (FFCMH), Mental Health America (MHA), and the National Alliance on Mental Illness (NAMI). The Bill of Rights sets forth a treatment standard that children, adolescents, and families should expect from mental-health providers. The item that best captures this expectation is: "children and their families should have access to a comprehensive continuum of care, based on their needs, including a full range of psychosocial, behavioral, pharmacological, and educational services, regardless of the cost" (AACAP 2008). Thus, it is expected that the psychiatric consultant, particularly in child psychiatry, use an integrated approach—in collaboration with both the treatment team and the children's families—regarding the decision-making processes.

In child and adolescent psychiatry as well as in pediatric consultation-liaison work, a shared decision-making role in the implementation of best-practice treatment plans can be complicated, especially when the medical or psychiatric illness occurs in a time of family system difficulty, such as divorce, legal trouble, financial strain, nontraditional lifestyles, death, etc.

Siblings

We wish to emphasize the importance a patient's siblings have in family systems. When working with families, the psychiatric consultant and treatment team often

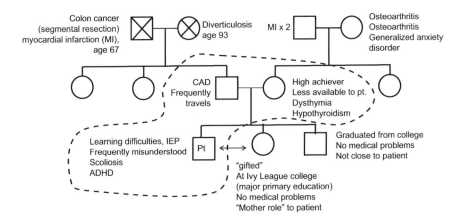

Fig. 4.2 A example genogram

overlook the significance of siblings. We have come a long way from Freud's belief that the sibling relationship is an extension of the Oedipus complex, with inherent competition and hostility (Freud 1924). Attachment theory research has highlighted the fact that positive sibling relationships can promote healthy and adaptive functioning (Stocker 1994; Tucker et al. 1999), while a history of negative sibling interactions can increase vulnerabilities and problem behaviors (Brody 2004; Snyder et al. 2005). Thus, failing to consider the importance siblings have in the treatment of patient and families in difficult psychiatric consultations can short change the treatment team, depriving its members of valuable medical and psychiatric information that may enhance the outcome. In the case of young siblings, attention should be given to their developmental level of understanding. They are frequently too immature to handle negative and distressing information and instead are shielded from the brunt of the loved one's illness. However, adult siblings may be able to provide the genetic linchpin needed for diagnostic formulations or the psychological linchpin needed to help the family reestablish cohesion.

The literature regarding organ transplants makes reference to the need to routinely perform a psychiatric evaluation of the recipient prior to surgery "to help determine the capacity to consent, the presence of psychiatric disorders, the suicidality, and the potential for self-care" (Mamah et al. 2004). Though there is also mention of the need for psychosocial evaluation of the parents of children with organ transplants (Stuber 2011), there is scant reference to assessing how the recipient may function within the context of their family system, and still less reference to the evaluation of immediate family members—including, for adults, a spouse or significant other. We recognize the importance of family systems and suggest that more attention be given to how family members, including siblings, function as a system when a member is diagnosed with a chronic serious illness.

The synergy created by all members can have positive influence in the patient's quality of life.

A House Divided: When Family Members Disagree About Treatment

Mr. Violet, a 65-year-old Caucasian, experiences a cerebrovascular accident involving his left middle cerebral artery and is acutely hospitalized and in a coma. During the course of his hospitalization, he requires mechanical ventilation, develops pneumonia and sepsis, for which broad-spectrum antibiotics are started, and he subsequently requires pressor support, which cannot then be weaned by his hospitalist. Mr. Violet's wife passed away 15 years prior to his illness, and at that time Mr. Violet moved to a small community so he could be close to his siblings. He has been active in community work and owns a small advertising firm. He has four successful adult children who live in other states. During the patient's stay, his hospitalist consults a neurologist. They communicate actively with the patient's family—his adult children and siblings—about the possibility of taking a "wait and see" approach, hoping that there could be a gradual recovery. This hope is based on their examinations, in spite of the fact that Mr. Violet's serial computed tomography scans reveal progression of the initial hemorrhage and that a consulting neurosurgeon believes that the prognosis is poor. There is a great deal of conflict among Mr. Violet's siblings, who are very religious, and his adult children, who are more pragmatic about what should be allowed to happen. There is also some confusion about his prognosis, as the hospitalist believes that Mr. Violet's recovery will take between 4 and 6 months and has requested that a social worker speak with the patient's children so they can begin the process of selecting a local extended-care facility. However, the neurosurgeon has openly stated there is little chance of recovery, and that the significant cerebral edema, with a real danger of brainstem herniation, indicates Mr. Violet will soon die. The family is in conflict. Mr. Violet's siblings feel they should be recognized as the immediate family, as they have lived in the same community and have been very close to him for the last 15 years. In short, Mr. Violet's siblings are hoping to "hang on longer" and, as a result of their religious beliefs, to avoid a Do Not Resuscitate order. Mr. Violet's adult children feel that the lack of life signs and their father's suffering are enough reason to allow him a peaceful death.

As may sometimes be the case in small communities, the consulting psychiatrist to the hospital is familiar with Mr. Violet, whom she has been treating for dysthymia for the last 3 years. The psychiatrist is well known within the community and is highly respected by the treating physicians involved in Mr. Violet's care. Because of her familiarity with the patient, she is asked to intervene in the conflict surrounding his care. She speaks to both sides of the family, reviewing their expectations and realities. Both are aware that Mr. Violet trusted his psychiatrist and feels that she is able to be objective. Though all the members of the family appreciate that the process of grief, mourning, and bereavement is necessary, each individual is in a different stage of the process. Mr. Violet's siblings have the fear of their own mortality reawakened by his inevitable death. The adult children are better able to let go, to rely on happy memories, and avoid any further suffering. Ultimately, Mr. Violet is allowed to die peacefully, and the family seems closer in recognizing the loss.

From an ethical standpoint, who had the capacity to make the final decisions regarding life support—whether it should be provided or withheld—needed to be decided? The patient's siblings, who lived in the same city, felt they had medical decision-making authority, as they knew him well and, in fact, one of them was with him when he had the cerebrovascular accident. However, the patient's adult children felt that, because they would be affected the most by a prolonged recovery, as they did not live in the community, they should have decision-making authority. The conflict was resolved when it became clear to all parties that their disagreements reflected their wish to have some control over issues of mourning, anger, and bereavement. Once the family members understood that they had control over their own emotions and that the realities of the patient's medical issues were beyond their control, they were able to plan Mr. Violet's funeral together. Although laws vary by state, most states ensure that immediate family members, when available, remain in charge of the end-of-life decisions. Usually laws are in place that require at least two physicians to declare a patient incapacitated.

4.6   Returning Home: Discharge from the Treatment Team's Care

Without a doubt, during the course of treatment of a patient's medical or psychiatric illness, especially if it requires a lengthy hospitalization, the treatment team serves as the patient and family's macrosystem or community. If a psychiatric consultation is involved, the consultant likely encourages the treatment team to allow for active participation with the families, with the goal of helping patients by containing many of their anxieties. When the treatment is completed and it is time to discharge the patient, the termination of the relationships established within the hospital or academic institution may bring forth a new set of unique complexities for all involved. When the relationships have been mature and the treatment has evolved as a partnership—positive use of permeable boundaries—with a successful outcome, many patients and families may have feelings of sadness but overall demonstrate gratitude and are happy to return their original environments. For others, however, it may be very frightening to separate from the treatment team, whom they have been engaged with for an extended period of time, even if their interactions were conflicted. For certain patients and families, the termination of care, which included daily meetings with team members for weeks and sometimes months, may be experienced as a significant loss to their system. This loss of the support of their macrosystem, to which they had adapted, brings forth anxieties about the return to the original microsystem, especially when the family knows they will be returning to a conflicted family system. Thus, a set of multilayered feelings and emotions may need to be addressed before the discharge in order to assure compliance with follow-up recommendations.

The unspoken anxieties that arise when a family anticipates the return to a microsystem with less support than they'd had during the course of treatment of the patient may take many forms. They may, for example, lead the patient or family to misinterpret the reasons for discharge and to feel as if they are being abandoned or asked to leave too soon. In situations where the course of treatment was encumbered by patient and family conflicts, the family may, prior to discharge, unconsciously undermine the positive results, making mistakes in the care of their loved one, hoping for an extension of the hospital stay. The family may "forget" to wear masks or to help the patient cough, ambulate, avoid certain foods, etc. The family, feeling connected and supported by the interactions with the treatment team, may create new problems to keep the team engaged. Because of these issues, the discharge phase is a period where treatment teams commonly request the help of a psychiatric consultant. The consultant will encourage the team to be sensitive to the fact that families who behave in this manner before discharge, finding negative ways of interaction, actually are fearful about returning to an environment that may not provide the medical or emotional security they have grown accustomed to. Schwab et al. (2013) capture this situation: "In the case of the medically ill child, in a hospital setting, when a parent reacts by taking further distance....not only is the child left more distressed but the parent will often seem to medical staff to be self-involved or otherwise insensitive to the child's needs as a bad parent rather than that the parent is trying to cope with an emotionally untenable situation." Some families may choose to triangulate with the patient against the treatment team; others may use the patient as a scapegoat and state that they believe the patient is "faking getting better; he/she just wants to go home," when indeed he or she has improved, and finally others may have permeable boundary problems and use these to sabotage the treatment by convincing the patient to refuse medication or treatment interventions when discharge is mentioned. The consulting psychiatrist can help the treatment team understand that the patient and family are hoping to avoid the anxiety-provoking feelings that a discharge brings. This will need to be addressed carefully so as to prevent for the treatment team from reacting counter-phobically by pressuring for discharge. In such cases, the treatment team may attempt to emphasize that inpatient hospitalization is no longer medically necessary and may begin to distance themselves from the patient and family's anxiety, rushing through rounds, etc.

4.7   Post Hospitalization Interventions

Post hospitalization follow-up should be seen as a continuation of the bio-psycho-social treatment plan initiated by the treatment team during the inpatient portion of the treatment. In this regard, it is important to recognize that the outpatient follow-up arrangements serve as a transitional object (Winnicott 1974) for the patient and family until they can regain the homeostasis that may have been lost during the hospitalization. For many, it will be helpful to know that they have follow-up appointments scheduled until the patient has fully recovered. This recovery usually parallels the family system's return to a "stable state." The family that had conflicts with the treatment team during the hospital stay will benefit from having the attending or primary resident of the team drop by, if possible, when they return for follow-up appointments. Though such a return may not be feasible for the attending physician or resident, who may remember the difficulties interacting with the family during the treatment of the patient, or because of a change in clinical rotation assignments, the psychiatric consultant can nevertheless emphasize that in spite of the conflicts, which may have been due to the family member's vulnerabilities with limited cognitive flexibility, temperamental challenges, and insecure attachment styles, they had established a trusting, albeit conflicted relationship with the treatment-team members. A brief hello and encouragement during the transfer of care to the outpatient team "you will be in good hands with my colleagues" can go a long way in preventing further conflicts for the patient and family.

The psychiatric consultant will benefit from reiterating to treatment teams that in order to have successful post-discharge interventions with the patient and family, it is necessary to have a great deal of flexibility in the scheduling of follow-up meetings. Although it's helpful to have all involved parties attend the appointment, this is unrealistic and should be carefully explained to the patient and family before discharge. When possible a member of the outpatient team should be encouraged to meet the patient and family prior to discharge. If the patient and family return to a microsystem that involves insecure attachment style, the fear of coming in for medical follow-ups will be reawakened. The patient and family may have not followed the recommendations reliably and, believing that "the doctors and nurses will not like us and will criticize us because we didn't do what we were supposed to," may intentionally "forget" the appointment, sadly risking the success of the outcome. Flexibility is essential in dealing with these kinds of anxious and conflicted families. One might, for example, contact them by phone to remind them of the appointment, allow alternate family members to be part of the outpatient visit, or conduct a follow-up by speaker phone.

4.8 Summary

An integrated approach, recognizing that a family system depends on all its members to find a degree of stable balance, is crucial for improved treatment outcomes. In order to provide a sense of hopefulness and purpose, the consultant must work toward understanding the fears and expectations of each family member. Perhaps the most challenging aspect for treatment teams working with difficult families is understanding and tolerating their anxieties, even if they are exhibited in the form of negative interactions. Families that experience anxiety and helplessness when their loved one is seriously ill may unconsciously resort to negative behaviors—triangulation, scapegoating, misuse of boundaries—in an effort to regain a sense of control over their environment. Treatment teams will benefit from seeking a psychiatric consultation to tease out how to best intervene and help the family participate in the treatment planning for their relative. As one of the author's mentors has said, "A negative interaction with families is better than no interaction at all. You at least have something to work with."

References

AACAP Bill of Rights (2008) http://www.aacap.org/galleries/govtaffairs/a_bill_of_rights_for_children_with_mental_health_disorders_and_their_families_2012.pdf
Afifi WA, Morgan SE, Stephenson MT et al (2006) Examining the decision to talk with family about organ donation applying the theory of motivated information management. Commun Monogr 73(2):188–215
Barker P (1992) Basic family therapy, 3rd edn. Oxford University Press, New York
Bowlby J (1999) Attachment, 2nd edition, attachment and loss, vol 1. Basic Books, New York
Brody GH (2004) Siblings' direct and indirect contributions to child development. Curr Direct Psychol Sci 13:124–126
Freud S (1924) The dissolution of the Oedipus complex. In: Strachey J (ed) The standard edition, vol 19. Hogarth Press, London, pp 172–179
Groves JE (1978) Taking care of the hateful patient. N Engl J Med 298(16):883–887
Guadagnoli E, Christiansen CL, DeJong W et al (1999) The public's willingness to discuss their preference for organ donation with family members. Clin Transplant 13:342–348
Hoffman L (1981) Foundations of family therapy. Basic Books, New York
Josephson AM (2008) Reinventing family therapy: teaching family intervention as a new treatment modality. Acad Psychiatry 32(5):405–413
Lvon B (1950) An outline of general system theory. Br J Philos Sci 1:134–165
Mamah D, Hong BA, Chapman WC (2004) Liver transplantation in a patient with undiagnosed bipolar disorder. Transplant Proc 36:2717–2719
McConville BJ, Delgado SV (2006) How to plan and tailor treatment: an overview of diagnosis and treatment planning. In: Klykylo WM, Kay J (eds) Clinical child psychiatry, second edition. Wiley, West Sussex (UK), pp 91–108
McGoldrick M, Gerson R, Shellenberger S (1999) Genograms: assessment and intervention, 2nd edn. W.W. Norton & Company, New York
Minuchin S (1974) Families and family therapy. Harvard University Press, Cambridge, MA
Minuchin S, Fishman HC (1981) Family therapy techniques. Harvard University Press, Cambridge, MA
Schwab A, Rusconi-Serpa S, Schechter DS (2013) Psychodynamic approaches to medically ill children and their traumatically stressed parents. Child Adolesc Psychiatr Clin North Am 22 (1):119–139
Snyder J, Bank L, Burraston B (2005) The consequences of antisocial behavior in older male siblings for younger brothers and sisters. J Fam Psychol 19:643–653
Stocker CM (1994) Children' s perceptions of relationships with siblings, friends, and mothers: compensatory processes and links with adjustment. J Child Psychol Psychiatry 35:1447–1459
Strous RD, Ulman AM, Kotler M (2006) The hateful patient revisited: relevance for 21st century medicine. Eur J Intern Med 17(6):387–393
Stuber ML (2011) Psychiatric issues in pediatric organ transplantation. Pediatr Clin North Am 58 (4):887–901
Tucker CJ, Updegraff KA, McHale SM et al (1999) Older siblings as socializers of younger siblings' empathy. J Early Adolesc 19:176–198

Turkel SB, Jacobson J, Munzig E et al (2012) Atypical antipsychotic medications to control symptoms of delirium in children and adolescents. J Child Adolesc Psychopharmacol 22 (2):126–130

Wachtel EF (1982) The family psyche over three generations: The genogram revisited. J Marital Fam Ther 8(35):335–343

Winnicott D (1966) The family and individual development. Basic Books, New York

Winnicott DW (1974) Playing and reality. Pelican Books, London

The Treatment Team

5

> *The good physician treats the disease; the great physician*
> *treats the patient who has the disease*
> —Sir William Osler, M.D. (1849–1919)

The goal of the consultant will also be to influence, over time, the treatment team's ability to use psychodynamic and attachment theory concepts in difficult cases. It is helpful for the psychiatric consultant to teach treatment-team members that the way patients and families perceive the team is a replay of a dynamic that's familiar to them and that they therefore unconsciously seek to recreate. In this chapter, we will describe a practical approach to common treatment team conflicts and present some useful psychodynamic (e.g., countertransference) and attachment theory-based concepts that may be used in difficult psychiatric consultations.

5.1 Evolution of the Treatment Team

In medicine, the treatment team consists of diverse individuals with unique skill sets who work together in the care of a particular patient or group of patients. The treatment team's task is to carefully examine the patient, documenting their presenting signs and symptoms, to formulate a working diagnosis, and then to implement and actively manage a best-practice treatment plan for the best reasonable outcome. The care-team model was developed in 1948 at New York's Montefiore Hospital, then later adopted at medical centers across the East Coast and, still later, throughout the USA (Wise et al. 1974). The effectiveness of treatment teams in academic and community medical centers has now been recognized for more than a half-century, and today many medical schools and residency training programs openly support the team-based approach to care, including formal instruction related to teamwork skills and collaboration with multilevel practitioners. Moreover, the treatment-team approach, which is now the dominant model for hospital-based health care, is understood to be a key factor in improving patients' outcomes as well as their safety (Leape et al. 2009), and is

S.V. Delgado and J.R. Strawn, *Difficult Psychiatric Consultations*,
DOI 10.1007/978-3-642-39552-9_5, © Springer-Verlag Berlin Heidelberg 2014

considered a critical aspect of inpatient health care by the American Hospital Association and The Joint Commission on Healthcare Accreditation (TJC 2010).

5.2   Anatomy of the Treatment Team

The treatment-team model typically seen in academic medical centers includes (1) an attending physician, (2) residents or fellows, (3) advanced-practice nurses, (4) nursing staff, (5) social workers, (6) medical students, (7) pharmacists, and may also include psychologists and/or dieticians. Depending on the primary specialty and function (e.g., surgical vs. nonsurgical, specialist vs. general medical), there is some degree of variability in the team's composition, but for a unit to function well, there must be a stable set of core members. The rules regarding leadership roles and duties are generally both spoken and unspoken. The treatment team may have formal daily meetings to review patients' progress and treatment recommendations, while other meetings, including those with the patient and family, may occur casually during bedside rounds. Recent thought has included the patient as part of the large treatment team, and as an active participant, he or she shares in the decision-making regarding their care. In short, treatment teams are practical and effective in formulating and implementing treatment recommendations, as well as monitoring them for efficacy (Wise et al. 1974).

There are situations in which the treatment team is utilized only for specific interventions, and the members of the team may not work together on a regular basis, as is the case with surgical teams when the surgeon, resident, operating-room nurse, and anesthesiologist rotate among many cases and teams. In the outpatient setting, the role of treatment team is more standardized, as in offices of pediatricians, ophthalmologists, and dentists. In these settings, due to the limited interactions between the family and the treatment team, a psychiatric consultation is rarely needed or even considered.

Characteristics of Treatment-Team Members

The members of a treatment team typically identify the person who will lead it, usually the senior physician, who then designates how the work will be divided, and how responsibilities will be assigned. This structure helps the patient and family know which team member is best equipped to address their questions or concerns about the diagnosis or treatment. As they have had similar professional career paths, members of a given treatment team have certain characteristics in common. They share the goal of working toward healing patients; they have been cognitively flexible when learning the importance of biopsychosocial issues; they have regularly used mature defense mechanisms in the academic and clinical spheres; they have a predominantly secure attachment style when interacting with colleagues and patients, with the ability to manage different opinions; they have had an easy/ flexible or slow-to-warm-up temperament that allows them to be active participants in learning and listening to patients; and they have the capacity to mentalize (Chap. 2), the ability to interpret behavior as meaningful and based on the mental states of oneself and of others, understanding what is expected of them by teachers and patients. In spite of the similarities among medical providers, however, there will be variability in areas of strength. For example, a colleague with a preference for working independently, with limited patient contact, pursues a career in radiology or pathology, while another colleague who excels at the complexities of diagnosis and treatment of medical conditions chooses to become an internist, and finally, a colleague who is readily able to mentalize, empathize, and is curious about how the human mind works, becomes a psychiatrist, child psychiatrist, psychologist, or social worker.

Having suggested some of the strengths within the members of a given treatment team, we will now review some of the possible areas of weakness. Although teams frequently and successfully struggle with patient and family conflicts, certain patients and families are able to elicit strong reactions from team members, which may interfere with the team's ability to provide the care expected. In this regard, members of treatment teams, however similar their goals, may be divided into two categories based on their ability to tolerate conflict, to allow for psychological closeness, and to mentalize. There are (1) practitioners who are skilled in working with patients but maintain psychological distance and avoid feelings of closeness and (2) practitioners who genuinely connect with their patients and are empathic and psychologically attuned to them.

Sympathy (Maintaining Psychological Distance)

Sympathy, unlike empathy, is the capacity to feel for someone's experience without necessarily being in their shoes (Irwin et al. 2008). Common examples of this are seen in everyday life when people send sympathy cards to family members and friends to express sorrow for either a difficult experience or a loss. When a treatment team offers or expresses sympathy to a patient or family, the recipient generally finds this approach supportive, although it may also be experienced by certain patients as insincere, patronizing, and judgmental. In the care of pediatric patients, sympathy often takes the form of reassurance. In such instances, the physician, resident, or nurse expresses sympathy to decrease their anxiety while examining the ear of a child with *otitis media* or when vaccinating a child who is frightened. As discussed in Chap. 2, when the patient and or family has an easy/flexible temperament, secure attachment style, and cognitive flexibility, the sympathy-based approach is well received and appreciated. However, this is often not the case in difficult psychiatric consultations, where the patient may have limited cognitive and affective flexibility, insecure attachment style, and a difficult/feisty temperament.

When treatment-team members who are accustomed to calming patients with sympathy interact with psychologically difficult patients, the patient's affective state can become difficult for the members to tolerate. For these patients or families, sympathy is not enough, as it leaves a degree of uncertainty and ambivalence about their care. The patient and/or family may feel isolated and, believing that team members are unable to grasp their state of mind, may begin to direct derogatory comments toward the team. The patient and family may then begin to challenge treatment recommendations, although they unconsciously are hoping for team members to contain their anxieties by making the disavowed negative projections of the self somewhat bearable and less frightening (Chap. 2). The treatment team, in turn, may unconsciously reject these projections, follow their inclination toward action over expression, and, in minimizing direct dialogue with patient and or family, distance themselves still further from the family's anxieties, although they continue working to provide the best-practice medical care to the patient. This will continue until there is a treatment impasse between patient, family, and the treatment team, at which point they will seek a psychiatric consultation.

Excessive sympathy may interfere with the objectivity required to deliver a diagnosis and recommend treatment for an illness that has a poor prognosis (Hojat et al. 2002). A physician who, out of sympathy, withholds negative information about the severity of the patient's illness to prevent the patient and family undue distress will quickly learn that this was not helpful and may lead to dysfunctional interactions among the patient, family, and treatment team. This situation, withholding negative information, can occur when the physician identifies with a patient who reminds him or her of their own close family member (age, name, and temperament) or of a prior patient who had a negative outcome.

A Treatment Team Misdirected by Feelings of Sympathy

A 24-year-old woman with an anorexia nervosa is admitted to the intensive care unit of the hospital as a result of a serious arrhythmia secondary to persistent hypokalemia and hypophosphatemia. As the patient improves and is stabilized, she asks to return home. The treatment team is sympathetic and supportive, even though the psychiatric consultant suggests it would be best if the patient was transferred to the psychiatric unit to prevent the risk of a serious relapse due to her denial of the severity of the eating disorder. The team leader offers sympathy to the patient, saying, "It must be frightening to be in the hospital, and I can see why you would want to go home," and observing that the patient is overall competent to make her own medical decisions, agrees with the discharge, withholding that she will most likely return, as her psychological state may prevent her from following through with treatment recommendations.

Empathy (Allowing Psychological Closeness)

Empathy reflects the ability to share the feelings that another person experiences, whether they be feelings of excitement or sadness. Webster's Unabridged Dictionary defines empathy as "the projection of one's own personality into the personality of another in order to understand the person better; ability to share in another's emotions, thoughts, or feelings" (Random House 2001).

As an example, when a parent consoles a child after he or she has lost in a competition he or she had spent months preparing for, the parent may draw on an understanding of how they themselves have been disappointed in the past. The shared feeling allows for the sense of having been "in their shoes," which is reflective of empathy and mentalizing abilities. The parent may constructively say, "I'm sorry you didn't win. I can imagine how frustrated you must be," with added reassurance that their relationship remains solid: "Let's celebrate all the hard work you put into this competition." Empathy is a blending of one person's past with another person's present, an overlapping of two emotional landscapes.

In the medical field, empathy is described as a multidimensional concept with variability among physicians due to differing personality styles, as is the case with sympathy. Hojat and colleagues (2002) developed the Jefferson Scale of Physician Empathy, a psychometrically validated tool that measures empathy in medical personnel. His tool was used with 1,007 physicians of multiple specialties in Philadelphia, and his results indicated that female physicians scored higher in empathy than their male counterparts. Psychiatrists, when controlled for gender, scored significantly higher than physicians specializing in anesthesiology, orthopedic surgery, neurosurgery, radiology, cardiovascular surgery, obstetrics and gynecology, and general surgery. Interestingly, Hojat observed no significant differences on empathy scores among physicians in psychiatry, internal medicine, pediatrics, emergency medicine, and family medicine. This is empirically consistent with the fact that treatment-team members who have the ability to sympathize, yet who have difficulty empathizing with patients' ambivalent and fearful feelings about their medical conditions, asked for psychiatric consultations more often. The request for consultation was primarily due to the conflicts that the patients and families had over the delivery of care from treatment teams. Cases frequently discussed by consultation-liaison psychiatrists at national conferences and in publications involve the psychiatric consultant encouraging the parties involved to have empathy for each other's dilemmas. In a review of the literature, Hojat et al. (2002) found that empathy is linked to many personal attributes in physicians, such as dutifulness, moral reasoning, good attitudes toward elderly patients, and that those physicians who employ empathy experience a reduction in malpractice litigation, greater patient satisfaction, better therapeutic relationships, and good clinical outcomes. Other research has provided support for what seems to be intuitively known—that female physicians express empathy and assume caring attitudes more than male physicians (Eagly and Steffen 1984; Reverby 1987).

An Unpopular Although Empathic Treatment Team

Revisiting the case described earlier in this chapter of the 24-year-old woman who is admitted to intensive care as a result of a serious arrhythmia secondary to persistent hypokalemia and hypophosphatemia due to the exacerbation of her eating disorder, we will describe how empathy may be used to approach the problems presented. When the patient improves and is stabilized, she asks the treatment team if she can return home. After private discussion, the team decides to transfer the patient to a medical floor or psychiatric unit, delivering this decision to the patient in an empathic manner that conveys their understanding of her dilemma, explaining that though she wishes to go home without further treatment for her chronic eating disorder, doing so would not be in her best interest. The treatment team shares with the patient that their goal is to help her prevent a potential relapse due to the severity of the eating disorder, stating, "We believe that it's too much of a burden for you to manage your illness outside of the hospital, and we want to help you avoid a relapse, even if you prefer to go home." The treatment team discusses with the patient whether they will need to sign "a hold" (involuntary psychiatric commitment) or whether she will accept a psychiatric treatment.

In the above example, the treatment team empathizes with the patient's anxiety and helps her to feel valued, without agreeing with her position. The team has served as the container for the patient's projections (Chap. 2). That is to say, the patient consciously feels that the treatment team represents her punitive self/object, when in fact they represent the disavowed and projected good self/object that she is unable to accept, as it would require insight about the seriousness of her illness. Her good self/object would recognize that her eating disorder is out of control and would welcome and benefit from following the treatment recommendations.

It is helpful for the psychiatric consultant to teach treatment-team members that the way patients and families perceive the team is a replay of a dynamic that's familiar to them (i.e., parent–child, family, marital conflicts, etc.) and that they therefore unconsciously seek to recreate. When the consultant works with the same treatment team over time, he or she may be in a position to familiarize members with psychodynamic and attachment theory concepts in the medical setting, thus improving the manner in which the team approaches patients.

The patient or family member with limited cognitive skills, who is temperamentally difficult/feisty, and has a history of a disorganized attachment style, will likely perceive the empathic physician as insensitive, pushy, and overbearing. Though the physician wishes to reassure them by presenting the medical information with certainty and conviction, the patient and family may feel they are being attacked and will respond with distancing behaviors—threatening to leave against medical advice, requesting a different physician or treatment team, and blaming the lead physician of the team for not treating them as well as they believe other patients have been treated. Although it is rare, the patient or family member with good cognitive skills, with an easy/flexible temperament, and with a history of a secure attachment style, may experience the empathic physician/treatment team— especially if he/she presents information in an overly intellectual manner, with a description of statistical data—as condescending and aloof. In both cases, the psychiatric consultant can help by educating team members about how to approach patients and families, based on their personality styles, which is as important as the best-practice treatment recommendations in improving outcomes.

5.3   Countertransference in the Psychiatric Consultant and the Treatment Team

Countertransference in the Psychiatric Consultant

Psychiatrists are familiar with the concept of countertransference and may easily recall the times in which they used the term. Until recently, countertransference was understood as an intrapsychic unconscious process in which there is a reawakening of conflicted childhood experiences evoked by the patient's transference to the psychiatrist. With the emergence of theories about intersubjectivity and affective attunement, we now believe that countertransference reactions do not exist in a vacuum and are best understood as a collection of the subjectivities between the patient and psychiatrist in the context of a here-and-now moment that creates a mutually shared experience. For example, a patient who receives the results of laboratory or diagnostic testing results and diagnosis of their illness reacts negatively, experiencing the physician delivering the information as insensitive and unempathic. The patient's reaction leads the physician to feel upset and does not allow time for discussion of the results and diagnosis. During the interaction, the physician, who may be tired or preoccupied with other patients, could be unaware of the fact that in the here-and-now moment with the patient, he or she actually came across as demanding. The patient, of course, has no way of knowing that the reasons for the physician's tone are not related to the patient him- or herself and thus they are unconsciously reminded of their demanding caregivers, which evoke a transference reaction to the forceful and unempathic physician. Consequently, when the physician experiences the patient as unappreciative, he or she may be unconsciously reminded of early childhood caregivers that were unappreciative of accomplishments, and a countertransference reaction to the patient transference may ensue. To take the analysis further, when theories of intersubjectivity are applied to the interactions between the patient and physician, the here-and-now moments that create a mutually shared experience of the two persons' "realities" can no longer be understood as solely in terms of transference and countertransference. The dance that occurs between two human subjective experiences, when mutually understood, can lead to great outcomes. When the shared experiences are opposed and complex, it leads to intertwined negative outcomes. If the physician has the capacity to take a step back and review with the patient what may have happened between them that led to the negative reactions, doing so can prevent conflicts from developing. Some physicians are more able than others to engage in this process. As Wachtel (2010) skillfully observed, "It is certainly true that each of us enters any interaction with certain proclivities, and that those proclivities have a strong bearing on how things proceed."

From the standpoint of consultative psychiatry, the astute consultant must remain vigilant about the countertransference feelings that may be elicited in response to the transferences by patients, families, and treatment teams. In order to prevent negative countertransference reactions and thus reduce the likelihood of conflict, the consultant will need to keep in mind what is known about the patient's, families and treatment team members' temperaments, their personality styles, their ability to mentalize, and their attachment style. However, it is important to remember that in contemporary theory, the psychiatric consultant's countertransference also contributes to consultative process interactions in here-and-now moments, as described in the case above.

Countertransference in the Treatment Team

Treatment-team members frequently have countertransference reactions to patients, families, and to psychiatric consultants. The members who are especially at risk are those with a limited ability to mentalize (Chap. 2).

When a team member has a countertransference reaction to a patient or their family, the psychiatric consultant can help by reminding the treatment team that the member engaged in the negative interaction need not remain at the center of the conflict. Diffusing the situation may be a simple matter of delegating tasks that involve patient contact to team members whose strengths are to better able to both process emotions and to serve as the container of patient's projections, as there may not be opportunities to transfer these patients to other treatment teams. The goal of the consultant will also be to influence, over time, the treatment team's ability to use psychodynamic and attachment theory concepts in difficult cases.

Dynamics to Which the Psychiatric Consultant May Need to Attend in Working with the Treatment Team

- The patient reminds the treatment team of a prior patient with negative outcome.
- The treatment team disagrees with patient or family regarding decisions as these contradicts their mission.
- Because of their action-oriented approach, the treatment team has difficulty tolerating the patient or his family's healthy ambivalence.
- Internal treatment team conflicts are exacerbated by the patient and/or family.
- Poor communication among treatment team members leads to inconsistent information being provided to patient and family.
- Avoidance discussion about the possibility of negative outcomes or death.

Perhaps one of the most difficult situations in consultative work is when treatment teams have countertransference reactions to the psychiatric consultant and their profession. This is common for non-psychologically minded individuals, and a treatment team made up of such individuals will have significant doubts about the consultant's treatment recommendations. Unfortunately, at times the psychiatric consultant may feel that "I know better than you" and get caught up in the treatment team's transference, which then elicits a negative countertransference reaction or a process of projective identification (Chap. 2). In doing so, the consultant may find him- or herself repeating the same conflicts they are hoping to resolve.

By understanding that the treatment team's reluctance in working collaboratively may be due to individual transference reactions, the consultant can avoid the interpersonal down spiral. When the treatment team as a whole has a negative reaction to the consultant, it is considered a group-dynamic phenomenon. Although such situations are beyond the scope of this book, the interventions that can best help with these impasses have been described in the family systems theory section (Chap. 4). When the consultant is expected to work with a particularly difficult treatment team repeatedly, it may be helpful, if the impasse persists, for the consultant to recognize his or her limitations and seek help from a colleague, who may provide a different perspective on the conflict.

The Noncompliant Pediatric Patient with a Chronic Medical Problem

Nikki, a 14-year-old girl with end-stage renal disease as a result of obstructive uropathy and a cloacal anomaly, has been on dialysis for two-and-a-half years. Her nephrologist refers her to an outpatient adolescent psychiatrist for "anxiety, difficulty with the dialysis staff and compulsive picking at a recurrent scalp wound" that has not "responded to" fluoxetine. During appointments with her psychiatrist, Nikki, a thin, ill-appearing girl, sits in a wheelchair, bundled in tattered sweatshirt and slippers, and speaks of not wanting to "go through with it all," referring to recent discussions of a kidney transplant. In these meetings she often references the pop musician Michael Jackson, whose life and recent death serve as a nidus for Nikki's sadness, anger, and curiosity. Her psychiatrist regularly sees Nikki in the dialysis unit and is able to observe how the dialysis staff become frustrated by the unexpected complications of Nikki's medical conditions and often express anger toward Nikki and her family, which inevitably makes Nikki psychologically regress. At one point, in the context of discussing finding "out-of-home placement" for Nikki to have better care than what they perceive she has been receiving from her mother, her nephrology team notes that it would be a "personal failure" if Nikki could not have a transplant.

She has required numerous hospitalizations and surgeries throughout her life. Her treatment consists of hemodialysis three times weekly, which she is expected to need until she receives her kidney transplant. She has difficulty complying with requests from the dialysis nurses, and because of this, the nephrology team asks for her admission to the inpatient psychiatric adolescent unit to better provide the needed treatment. The nephrology team also requests guidance about how to improve Nikki's compliance with her medications, as they feel her noncompliance has led to medical complications delaying her transplant: osteomyelitis in her scalp, difficult-to-control hypertension, and abnormal electrolytes. Until these are resolved, her candidacy as a kidney recipient is on hold. Her treatment team had hoped that the patient would be more active in her self-care, thereby "speeding up her readiness for a transplant." The delay has seemed especially long for her nephrology team, given the fragile state of Nikki's health, although the treatment team has also felt a strong sense of urgency. Typically, in working with nephrology patients in need of kidney transplants, a crucial step is finding the appropriate donor at a time of optimal health in the recipient. In Nikki's case, her living donor is to be her mother, cleared by the transplant team.

Nikki worries about her scalp wound and shares that her picking increases when she is nervous, which makes her distraught because she cannot stop: "Maybe I'm going insane. Maybe I'm crazy because I keep picking my body." Her picking behavior noticeably worsens following the termination of home health care services. The nephrology team sees Nikki's mother as being neglectful and requests foster-home placement. The foster-care services end within 3 days, when the social services case manager notes that Nikki "picked her scalp wound nonstop" in the foster home. Upon Nikki's return home, her mother— sensitive to the situation they are in—voluntarily agrees to keep their case open with social services, because "the case manager can help when we need transportation or when Nikki needs more than what I can give her." The nurse responsible for home health services shares with the nephrology team that Nikki's mother uses the services well and that it has allowed her to be "a mother" rather than "a nurse." This shift in the system has lead to significant positive changes within the family and the patient. Thus, the relatively abrupt termination of the home health care relationship creates a significant source of anxiety and sadness for Nikki and her family.

Upon Nikki's admission to the adolescent inpatient psychiatric unit, the psychiatrist and his treatment team meet regularly with the nephrology team and soon realize that the most difficult issue for the team is not her behavior but rather her having recently begun to speak about her wish to die, which is at odds with the nephrology team's wish that she receive a kidney transplant. Her wanting to openly share her feelings and dilemmas is difficult and frustrating for her mother and her nephrology team. Fortunately, Nikki has an outpatient psychiatrist, who also is her psychotherapist and psychodynamically trained. During her psychiatric admission, he would meet in her room during the regular psychotherapy appointment times in order to maintain predictability in this aspect of her life. The outpatient psychiatrist has been a stable figure for Nikki, as he has been providing psychotherapy and medication management for nearly a year. Nikki has openly spoken with her psychiatrist and the psychiatric nursing staff about not being afraid to die and has shared her ambivalence about going through with the kidney transplant. She also shares with her outpatient psychiatrist her fantasies about Michael Jackson's death and how peaceful he must have been when he "fell asleep for the last time." However, as proof of her ambivalence, she talks about her anger at Michael Jackson's physician, whom she describes as having "allowed him to die," something frequently discussed at that time in the news media. These discussions are emotionally difficult for her outpatient psychiatrist. Though he understands them to be a safe displacement of her fears, they lead to feelings of countertransference, specifically, his wanting to stop discussing death fantasies and speak of happier matters. The patient's ambivalence is difficult for him to tolerate, even though he knows it is necessary and requires time to work through. The patient's family and her nephrology team also begin to elicit feelings of countertransference in the outpatient psychiatrist, as they express concern that Nikki is talking about death "too much in therapy" and fear it will increase her depressive symptoms and lead her to want to "give up." The nephrology team asks Nikki's mother and the inpatient psychiatric team to consider changing her outpatient psychiatrist, "to get a fresh look at her needs and maybe to change her medications."

The inpatient psychiatric treatment-team suggests that it would be in Nikki's best interest, not to be informed of her mother's and the nephrology team's conflicted feelings about her outpatient psychiatrist. Nikki's psychiatrist is supported by the inpatient team, who are aware that to help Nikki with her ambivalence, it is necessary to allow the expression and working through of her fears. Her psychiatrist is also aware that "those [patients] who chose hemodialysis showed a tendency to adopt an image-distorting defense style" (Hyphantis et al. 2010), and this is consistent with Nikki's personality traits and her behavior of excessively picking her scalp during the course of treatment. The outpatient psychiatrist is invited to participate in the inpatient treatment-team meetings that include Nikki's mother, the nephrology team, and her case manager. During the course of her hospitalization, the psychiatric staff—which is used to adolescents initially rejecting help—approach Nikki with a sense of calm and, in doing so, facilitate healthier interactions with those who care about her outcome. Nikki learns to accept the new sense of mutuality with the psychiatric team, which allows her to achieve the goal of feeling comfortable accepting assistance in her difficult situation. The psychiatric staff is able to help Nikki recognize that she can be a partner in giving suggestions to the nephrology team about interventions that might work for her, which, rather than focusing on their frustration (a common reaction among medical personnel when children resist care), conveys that they are championing Nikki wishes to succeed.

The psychiatric staff has daily communication with the nephrology team, reassuring them of her progress emotionally and how she has improved in her willingness to participate in the treatment milieu. The nephrology team has difficulty accepting her improvement and begins to wonder whether Nikki is "pretending" when participating in the milieu, as if the psychiatric staff's comments are not accurate.

With regard to the renal transplantation, Nikki's mother often shares that Nikki does not want a transplant, is tired of dialysis, and does not want to continue. Nikki's mother continues to relay that Nikki feels like a burden to the family. To address the multiple aspects of her care and the myriad reactions to transplantation, a care conference is arranged involving Nikki's inpatient and outpatient psychiatrists, her nephrologist, dialysis nurse, case worker, and her mother. The nephrology team comes to the conference hoping those involved can find more effective ways to engage Nikki in treatment, as they have become focused on her poor past compliance. Her primary dialysis nurse has been directing her frustrations toward the patient's mother and the psychiatric treatment team, as she believes they have been encouraging Nikki's feelings of hopelessness. Although difficult for most at the care conference to hear, suggestions are made about considering palliative care to help Nikki with her thoughts and feelings about death and her quality of life. The inpatient and outpatient psychiatrists quickly realize that any attempt by the psychiatric treatment team to explain the current admission in psychological terms, associated with the sadness and fear over the loss of her close home-health nurse, will be deflected by the nephrology team, who insist that she had not been receiving adequate support from her mother and her outpatient psychiatrist, which to them explains the reason for her noncompliance. During the course of the care conference, it is discussed that Nikki has received hemodialysis for 7 years and says she hates getting up in the morning. She is ambivalent about wanting a kidney transplant and states, "Sometimes I just feel like cussing." Nikki continues to improve on the psychiatric unit and attends programming regularly. At the time of her discharge, Nikki is less angry, more able to express her frustration with the treatment team, and is both less anxious and less ambivalent about living.

This case illustrates many difficult aspects of patient autonomy in a pediatric setting, where decisions regarding treatment are usually the purview of the parents and the psychiatric consultant. The complexities revolve around what tools should be employed when the best-practice care is not accepted by a patient. The psychiatric consultant approaching a case such as Nikki's, in which there is profound disagreement among treatment-team members, may have several important tasks (Table 5.1). First, the consultant must teach and model the ability to tolerate ambiguity regarding outcomes. Second, he or she would do well to recognize that the treatment team may feel compelled to find "answers" in an effort to decrease their anxiety. Third, and most important, the consultant must openly and explicitly acknowledge the conflict among team members over the possibility of the patient's death. In doing so, the psychiatric consultant creates a potential space in which these conflicts can be "aired out" as opposed to "acted out." Finally, the consultant needs to recognize the "scape-goat" role, into which the patient can be cast by treatment teams (see Chap. 4). When the patient is placed in this role, the treatment team is distanced from conflict, though sadly with a false sense of safety and accomplishment, as their behavior can adversely influence outcome.

Diagnostic Formulation and Interventions for Nikki (Table 5.1).
The Patient. Nikki has had serious medical difficulties since birth, and many of her early days were spent in the institutional setting of the hospital. These experiences profoundly influenced the development of her view of both self and others, and these distorted perceptions were compounded by her innate limited cognitive skills. Moreover, her temperament is difficult/feisty, which surprisingly has helped her survive the many medical treatments needed throughout her life, including more than 50 surgical procedures. Her immature defense mechanisms have also been largely helpful in that they've facilitated the management of constant anxiety over her health since birth. For Nikki, there is no

Table 5.1 The noncompliant pediatric patient with a chronic medical problem

	Patient before diagnosis	Patient after diagnosis	Family before diagnosis	Family after diagnosis	Treatment team members	Suggested consultant's intervention
Observed cognition	Limited		Good		*Inflexible*	• Helps treatment team members recognize their own difficulty tolerating the young patient's ambivalence, despair and possible poor outcome
Observed temperament	*Difficult/feisty*	*Difficult/feisty*	*Easy/flexible*	*Easy/flexible*	*Difficult/feisty*	• After noting that the main change in temperament occurred in the treatment team, the consultant helps them to recognize that their reactions may represent the fear that they may not be able to provide this young patient's a kidney transplant
Observed defense mechanisms	Stressful life since birth	*Immature*	Stressful life after birth of child		*Immature*	
Observed attachment style	Anxious		Anxious	Anxious	*Anxious*	• Encourages the treatment team to establish an alliance with Nikki's mother as she has been the stable support for Nikki through her struggles
Family	*The fragile child*		Supportive Stabilizer		*Triangulation*	• Considers involvement with the hospital ethics committee or a case conference to help the treatment team reflect on realistic expectations for this patient • Helps the treatment team understand the importance of the patient's therapist with regard to nonmalfecience and autonomy
Ethics	*Autonomy vs. beneficence*				*Autonomy vs. benefecince* *Autonomy vs. nonmalfecience* *treatment team suggests* *changing therapist*	

The table may be used to succinctly identify and assess the areas that require action by the psychiatric consultant in complex psychiatric consultation. It permits a careful and practical multidimensional assessment of the patient, his or her family and the treatment team and will facilitate interventions that will allow the consultant to collaborative with all parties, with the best interests of the patient in mind. In the table, we have used *italics* text to indicate relevant changes (e.g., pre-diagnosis and post-diagnosis), which may be the focus of clinical attention "before diagnosis" and "after diagnosis," as her psychological development has been concomitant with a series of complicated medical dilemmas.

Intervention by Psychiatric Consultant. The consulting psychiatrist reassures Nikki that her work with her outpatient psychiatrist/psychotherapist—with whom she feels understood and free to speak openly about her feelings and fears (i.e., her wish to die, her ambivalence about undergoing kidney transplantation, and her hope for a better life)—will be supported.

The Family. Nikki's mother is a resilient single parent who has served as a stabilizing figure for her daughter and has been active in the decision-making process when needed. She has learned to use her own family, case managers, home health workers, and her daughter's psychiatrist/psychotherapist as her support system.

Intervention by Psychiatric Consultant. The consultant provides support and listens empathically to Nikki's mother, helping to bridge what seems a negative interaction between the nephrology team and Nikki's hospital-based psychiatrist/psychotherapist.

The Treatment Team. Using Table 5.1, the psychiatric consultant may quickly recognize that the nephrology team, not Nikki or her mother, has undergone the most changes. The nephrology team has a history of good rapport with the patient and her mother, yet because of the physical and psychological changes within Nikki, and because of her "resistance to treatment," they began to scapegoat her, her psychiatrist/psychotherapist, and her mother. That is, they project their anxieties about Nikki's outcome onto others without recognizing their contribution to the conflict. This leads the team to become inflexible regarding psychological, family, and system matters, and they request a psychiatric consultation with hope that the patient, mother, and psychiatrist/psychotherapist will be made to "follow our recommendations," adding a tacit ultimatum: "Otherwise, we will request that the patient be removed from her mother and see a different psychiatrist/psychotherapist who can get her to take care of herself and not talk about death." As the table illustrates, there is a shift in the treatment team toward less cognitive flexibility, more difficulty relating with others, use of immature defense mechanisms, scapegoating, and a desire to triangulate with the psychiatric team.

Intervention by Psychiatric Consultant. The psychiatric consultant first establishes an alliance with the nephrology team and later uses his expertise to teach and model the ability to tolerate ambiguity regarding outcome, encouraging the team not to make the medical goals personal and to seek "answers" as a way of decreasing their anxiety. The team desires control over the situation: "Once we decide they need a transplant, we do not talk with the patient about not wanting to go through it. It is up to us." In response, the psychiatric consultant explicitly acknowledges the conflict surrounding the patient's talk of refusing the transplant, which allows her to feel like an active shareholder in her future (Suthanthiran and Storm 1994; Tonelli et al. 2011). The consultant may also be seen as "containing" the team's anxiety over Nikki's poor prognosis and the potential failure of conventional treatments, in spite of their clinical determination. The concept of "containing" a person's anxiety is rooted in the British psychoanalyst Wilferd Bion's (1897–1979) theory from the 1940s, which posits that the therapist is a container and, in this role, both holds and provides a thinking function so that the projection may be safely processed and reintrojected by the patient (Ferro 2005). In this regard, the psychiatric consultant contains and "digests" the treatment team's anxiety, but recognizes that his interventions only temporarily shift the observed attachment style. A more enduring change in attachment style occurs at an individual level and requires a new, nurturing, and stable environment or a psychotherapeutic process. In this case, the consultant allows the treatment-team members to continue to use an anxious attachment style (Chap. 2) with mature defense mechanisms (Chap. 2).

Ethics. This case illustrates the conflict between autonomy and beneficence in a pediatric setting within the context of an overly anxious treatment team fearful of a negative outcome.

Intervention by Psychiatric Consultant. The consultant works with the treatment team to help them better understand the role of autonomy with regard to the patient versus beneficence, which has been the primary guiding ethical principle prior to the psychiatric consultation.

The Psychotherapist Becomes a Member of Treatment Team

The role of empathic attunement experienced in the unique setting/structure of psychotherapy emerges as the single critical variable for a successful outcome
                                                                —Jeremy Spiegel (2000)

On occasion, the patient may have a psychotherapist before the diagnosis of a serious medical or psychiatric illness. When this is the case, the psychotherapist may be asked, by the patient or by the treatment team, to become a member of the team or to serve as a psychiatric consultant in difficult situations. Though this may bring a new set of complicating factors, it can also provide myriad positive opportunities as the psychotherapist has intimate information about the patient and family before the medical issues heightened feelings of vulnerability and anxiety. Before agreeing to collaborate, the psychotherapist will need to clarify with the patient and family what information they are comfortable having shared with the treatment team and other medical providers. In fact, a written consent should be obtained and documented in the patient's electronic medical record. It is also important to discuss whether the patient or family wishes the psychotherapist to communicate with the treatment team only when the patient is present or if it is acceptable to meet with the team in the absence of the patient or family.

When the psychotherapist working with a patient grappling with chronic medical illness is asked to intervene and to help the family as well, it can be challenging, as family conflicts may be part of the therapeutic process being addressed. The close relationship and rapport between psychotherapist and patient may need to shift, and the patient may struggle with allowing the psychotherapist to communicate actively with the family and treatment team, even though the patient finds this helpful. The psychotherapist will need to be attentive to many issues, first and foremost, his or her loyalty to the patient's confidentiality, as well as to the risk of countertransference feelings. Furthermore, it is very helpful for the patient to know that after the medical treatment is complete; their psychotherapist will continue to be a close ally during their recovery process. In more common situations, when a patient or family members do not have a psychotherapist prior to hospital stays, treatment teams who are sensitive to the nature of serious or chronic medical illnesses may recommend that the patient and family seek psychotherapy after the diagnosis. Such action is strongly encouraged, as treatment outcomes are greatly improved (Berry et al. 2013; Harman et al. 2005; Lask and Matthew 1979; Svedlund et al. 1983).

5.4   Summary

In addition to providing standard consultation (e.g., clarifying diagnosis, providing psychopharmacologic recommendations, ordering diagnostic studies), an added goal of the consultant may be to influence, over time, the treatment team's ability to use psychodynamic and attachment theory concepts in difficult cases. It is helpful for the psychiatric consultant to teach treatment-team members that the way patients and families perceive the team is a replay of a dynamic that's familiar to them and that they therefore unconsciously seek to recreate. When the consultant works with the same treatment team over time, he or she may be in a position to familiarize members with psychodynamic and attachment theory concepts in the medical setting, thus improving the manner in which the team approaches patients. Treatment-team members frequently have countertransference reactions to patients, families, and to psychiatric consultants. The members who are especially at risk are those with a limited ability to mentalize. However, it is important to remember that in contemporary theory, the psychiatric consultant's countertransference also contributes to consultative process interactions in here-and-now moments.

References

Berry LL, Rock BL, Smith Houskamp B et al (2013) Care coordination for patients with complex health profiles in inpatient and outpatient settings. Mayo Clin Proc 88(2):184–194
Eagly AH, Steffen VJ (1984) Gender stereotypes stem from the distribution of women and men into social roles. J Personal Soc Psychol 46:735–754
Ferro A (2005) Bion: theoretical and clinical observations. Int J Psychoanal 86:1535–1542
Harman JS, Edlund MJ, Fortney JC et al (2005) The influence of comorbid chronic medical conditions on the adequacy of depression care for older. J Am Geriatr Soc 53(12):2178–2183

Hojat M, Gonnella JS, Nasca TJ et al (2002) Physician empathy: definition, components, measurement and relationship to gender and specialty. Am J Psychiatry 159(9):1563–1569

Hyphantis T, Katsoudas S, Voudiclari S (2010) Ego mechanisms of defense are associated with patients' preference of treatment modality independent of psychological distress in end-stage renal disease. Patient Prefer Adherence 2(4):25–32

Irwin K, Mcgrimmon T, Simpson B (2008) Sympathy and social order. Soc Psychol Q 71 (4):379–397

Lask B, Matthew D (1979) Childhood asthma: a controlled trial of family psychotherapy. Arch Dis Child 54(2):116–119

Leape L, Berwick D, Clancy C et al (2009) Transforming healthcare: a safety imperative. Qual Saf Health Care 18(6):424–428

Random H (2001) Random House Webster's unabridged dictionary, 2nd edn. Random House, New York, NY

Reverby SS (1987) A caring dilemma: womanhood and nursing in historical perspective. Nurs Res 36(1):5–11

Spiegel J, Severino SK, Morrison NK (2000) The role of attachment functions in psychotherapy. J Psychother Pract Res 9(1):25–32

Suthanthiran M, Strom TB (1994) Renal transplantation. N Engl J Med 331(6):365–376

Svedlund J, Ottoson J, Sjodin I et al (1983) Controlled study of psychotherapy in irritable bowel syndrome. Lancet 2(8350):589–592

The Joint Commission (2010) Comprehensive accreditation manual for hospitals: the official handbook. Joint Commission Resources, Oak Brook, IL

Tonelli M, Wiebe N, Knoll G et al (2011) Systematic review: kidney transplantation compared with dialysis in clinically relevant outcomes. Am J Transplant 11(10):2093–2109

Wachtel PL (2010) One-person and two-person conceptions of attachment and their implications for psychoanalytic thought. Int J Psychoanal 91:561–581

Wise H, Beckhard R, Rubin I et al (1974) Making health teams work. Ballinger Publishing, Cambridge, MA

Ethical and Medicolegal Issues

6

> *Good people do not need laws to tell them to act responsibly,*
> *while bad people will find a way around the laws*
> —Plato (427–347 bc)

This chapter will address ethical and medicolegal issues that are particularly relevant to complex psychiatric consultations and that create special challenges for the consulting psychiatrist working with both pediatric (Ascherman and Rubin 2008) and adult populations (Arras and Steinbock 1998; Gutheil et al. 2005). Ethical and medicolegal concerns are common sources of anxiety, estrangement, and conflict among the involved parties and may delay or complicate a patient's treatment. Below, we will briefly review the four basic ethical principles—*autonomy*, *nonmaleficence*, *beneficence*, and *justice*—and will then describe specific ethical considerations relevant to consultation or care for the complex psychiatric patient, including confidentiality, privilege, and dual relationships. We will also review relevant medicolegal issues, including consent and assent, limits of confidentiality, and involuntary hospitalization.

6.1 A Brief History of Ethics in Medicine

As early as 500 bc, during the era of Hippocrates (Fig. 6.1), Greek physicians began to establish ethical codes, which were written officially as the Hippocratic Oath (Table 6.1, Edelstein 1967; Majumdar 1995). Widely used by medieval physicians, this oath emphasized the physician's power to heal and the need for the physician to be free of malice and aggression. Furthermore, the Hippocratic Oath enumerated the ethical obligations and duties that the physician had to the patient and created an expectation of confidentiality. Reflecting on the Hippocratic Oath, the sociologist Margaret Mead (1901–1978) noted that "the code clearly separated the physician from the sorcerer or shaman who had the power to both harm and cure" (Schetky 2007). Over the last two millennia, there have been significant advances in the understanding of ethical principles and additional "codes of ethics," including some

S.V. Delgado and J.R. Strawn, *Difficult Psychiatric Consultations*,
DOI 10.1007/978-3-642-39552-9_6, © Springer-Verlag Berlin Heidelberg 2014

Fig. 6.1 Hippocrates
National Library of Medicine

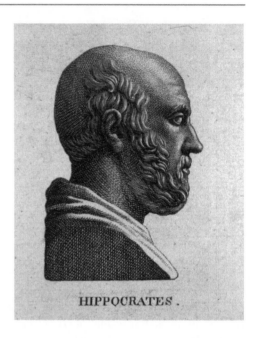

Table 6.1 The Hippocratic oath

I swear by Apollo, the healer, Asclepius, Hygieia, and Panacea, and I take to witness all the gods, all the goddesses, to keep according to my ability and my judgment, the following oath and agreement.
To consider dear to me, as my parents, him who taught me this art; to live in common with him and, if necessary, to share my goods with him; to look upon his children as my own brothers, to teach them this art; and that by my teaching, I will impart a knowledge of this art to my own sons, and to my teacher's sons, and to disciples bound by an indenture and oath according to the medical laws, and no others.
I will prescribe regimens for the good of my patients according to my ability and my judgment and never do harm to anyone.
I will give no deadly medicine to any one if asked, nor suggest any such counsel; and similarly I will not give a woman a pessary to cause an abortion.
But I will preserve the purity of my life and my arts.
I will not cut for stone, even for patients in whom the disease is manifest; I will leave this operation to be performed by practitioners, specialists in this art.
In every house where I come I will enter only for the good of my patients, keeping myself far from all intentional ill-doing and all seduction and especially from the pleasures of love with women or men, be they free or slaves.
All that may come to my knowledge in the exercise of my profession or in daily commerce with men, which ought not to be spread abroad, I will keep secret and will never reveal.
If I keep this oath faithfully, may I enjoy my life and practice my art, respected by all humanity and in all times; but if I swerve from it or violate it, may the reverse be my life.

that speak directly to the ethical dilemmas of psychiatrists, such as the American Psychiatric Association Code of Ethics, the American Medical Association Principles of Ethics with Special Annotations Applicable to Psychiatry (American Psychiatric Association 2009), and the American Academy of Child and Adolescent Psychiatry Code of Ethics (2009).

6.2   The Ethical Principles

Autonomy

The term *autonomy* originates from the Greek roots "self" and "rule" and, when applied to the medical sphere, registers a patient's right to self-determination. This principle derives from the societal respect for an ill individual who is making an informed decision regarding treatment (or refusing treatment). Further, the concept of autonomy underlies the increased use of advance directives (written instructions, such as a living will or durable power of attorney, which provide direction if the patient's decision-making capacity is impaired) in today's practice of medicine, including psychiatry. As will be discussed later in this chapter, the psychiatric consultant is frequently asked to evaluate a patient's capacity to make decisions regarding treatment, especially as the cognitive processes underlying that capacity can be impaired by various neuropsychiatric conditions (e.g., dementia, delirium, intoxication, schizophrenia, etc.). As such, this evaluation directly relates to the ethical principle of autonomy. However, unless a clear advance directive from the patient, prior to illness, exists, he will generally be treated in accordance with his best interests, an ethical issue relating to the balance of *autonomy* and *beneficience* (discussed below).

Beneficence

Beneficence refers to the physician's obligation to help others and to promote the patient's welfare. In other words, this ethical pillar directs treating physicians, treatment-team members, and consultants to act in the best interests of their patients, and considers that patients—because of medical or psychiatric conditions—represent a particularly vulnerable group who rely on the physician's guidance. This principle further requires physicians to "put the interests of their patients ahead of their own or those of third parties, such as insurers or managed care organizations" (Pantilat and Lo 2005).

Nonmaleficence

This ethical principle is derived from the Latin *primum non nocere*, or *first, do no harm*, and stems from the Hippocratic Oath, which states, "I will use treatment to help the sick according to my ability and judgment, but I will never use it to injure or wrong them" (Schetky 2007). Nonmaleficence serves to remind physicians and treatment-team members to carefully consider the adverse effects associated with treatments and is commonly seen as a corollary to *beneficence*.

Justice

Simply put, justice guides the physician in how to treat "similarly situated patients similarly and [to] allocate resources fairly" (Pantilat and Lo 2005). This principle ensures that patients receive equal care regardless of demographic, sociocultural, economic, and psychological differences. To assure that actions are "just," interventions should be based on standards of care that can be applied to society as a whole. This principle is also of relevance in our current economy, as many facilities and hospitals face limited healthcare resources, bringing to bear the necessity of practicing cost-effective medicine.

Confidentiality and Privacy

Confidentiality is of paramount importance in difficult psychiatric consultations. In the modern medical center, however, there are varying levels of confidentiality and potentially conflicting edicts related to its enforcement. At present, both federal and state laws protect the privacy and confidentiality of medical information. To this end, the Health Insurance Portability and Accountability Act standards were established in 1996 and implemented in 2003 as the Privacy Rule (HIPAA 1996). The Privacy Rule assures that individuals' health information is properly protected while it allows for the flow of health information needed to provide quality health care. The rule is designed to be flexible as well as comprehensive.

Healthcare providers have a profound responsibility to safeguard confidentiality. This principle is obliquely related to *autonomy* and *beneficence*, and has special importance for the psychiatric consultant and treatment team working with the complex psychiatric patient, as will be discussed in the next section. It is worth noting that, under some circumstances, this principle may be violated when legally required (e.g., child or elder abuse, or imminent danger relating to suicidal ideation or homicidal ideation/intent).

Regarding the difficult psychiatric consultation, there are three important aspects related to confidentiality that merit additional discussion, as they may create confusion among patients, treatment teams, and psychiatric consultants.

First, within the modern medical center and among treatment-team members, there are situations in which strict confidentiality limits are attenuated in the interest of patient care. In most academic centers, a patient's confidential medical information, if part of their record, may be shared with the treatment team and psychiatric consultant without obtaining specific consent from the patient or their family. As an example, a patient who is admitted for treatment of a community-acquired pneumonia (CAP) may be asked by team members about the status of his chronic headaches and depression, which the team discovered in reviewing the notes from the patient's electronic medical record (EMR).

Second, if the patient has been involved in psychotherapeutic work prior to the psychiatric consultation, confidentiality of psychotherapy material is heightened, and special protections are in place. Just as there are circumstances in which strict confidentiality seems to be relaxed to permit collaboration among treatment-team members, there are times when efforts must be made to fortify the patient's confidentiality. For the psychiatric consultant, the most common example involves the psychotherapeutic process. Those providing psychotherapy generally keep documentation separate from the primary medical record (whether in electronic or paper form), and these portions of the record should only be accessed after obtaining specific written informed consent of the patient. The goal of this "accentuated" confidentiality, albeit in a limited circumstance, is to protect the patient within the frame of a psychotherapeutic relationship. For example, a patient in psychotherapy who is working with his hospital-affiliated psychiatrist to understand resentment and anger toward close family members may later need the support of these family members. If the treatment team were to review the psychotherapy notes with the intent of knowing as much as possible about the patient, they may notice the conflict with certain family members and inadvertently disclose their anxiety about including the family members in the decision-making process. To prevent this, in some institutions, the EMR program may have a specific section that is confidential and can only be accessed by the person who made the entry or by a provider from the same department. This is particularly important when the patient is actively working on prior psychological trauma or legal matters during the psychotherapy process.

Third, when a treatment-team member or the psychiatric consultant has a prior relationship with the patient or family member outside of the treatment relationship, this has profound implications, not only for confidentiality, but also for boundaries and boundary perceptions. Confidentiality difficulties may arise for the psychiatric consultant or treatment team if a patient or family member is a colleague, friend, relative, or someone who is known to the provider outside of the treatment relationship. In these circumstances, it is critical to define the treatment relationship and to be cognizant of unspoken expectations regarding treatment, contact (e.g., cell phone communication, email, stopping by the house), and confidentiality (e.g., discussions at church or in the neighborhood). The consultant working with a patient who has a preexisting relationship with a treatment-team member should be alert to a patient's tendency to consent to a treatment—because of the preexisting relationship—which he or she might otherwise question. Moreover, the psychiatric consultant should look for opportunities to discourage boundary blurring between treater and friend or treater and relative, which will permit both the patient and the team member to interact more freely.

6.3   Medicolegal Issues

In addition to ethical issues, physicians in treatment teams are also bound by the medicolegal matters governing the discipline (Wecht 2005). It is important to have a working understanding of the interface between medicine, psychiatry, and the law, which of necessity has evolved to protect medically or mentally-ill individuals, as well as their families, from irresponsible acts occurring during their care (Levenson 2013; Simon et al. 2005; Swanepoel 2009). For the psychiatric consultant, the most common medicolegal issues will involve: (1) determination of decision-making capacity, (2) informed consent, and (3) involuntary hospitalization, which are described in the subsequent sections.

Determination of Decision-Making Capacity

The ability to consent to treatment is predicated on the patient having what is commonly referred to as "decision-making capacity." Importantly, decision-making capacity, which is a global determination and may fluctuate, is different from competency; the latter is determined by the court, while the former can be determined by most licensed physicians (Appelbaum 2007; Appelbaum and Grisso 1988). Because various factors that can influence decision-making capacity are related to both medical and psychological processes, consulting psychiatrists are often involved in the assessment.

In determining capacity, there are four key processes that must be intact: (1) communication, (2) understanding, (3) appreciation, and (4) the patient's ability to provide rational reasons for his or her decisions. All of these elements must be present for the patient to be deemed as having the capacity to give or withhold consent. With regard to communication, the patient must be able to freely express their treatment choice. In terms of the second component, understanding, the patient must be able to recall information shared during treatment discussions by medical providers. In assessing understanding, the consultant should pay particular attention to disorders affecting memory and processing information (e.g., dementia, learning disorders, intellectual disability, and delirium). The third element, appreciation, involves the patient's ability to "identify the illness, treatment options, and likely outcomes as things that will affect him or her directly" (Appelbaum 2007; Mahajan et al. 2008). Finally, the patient must demonstrate having clear, rational reasons for his or her decisions. This component is often influenced by psychological factors like anxiety, as well as psychiatric processes including depression and psychosis. In recent years, some clinicians have advocated the use of standardized approaches to determining capacity—specifically the Mini Mental Status Examination, or MMSE (Crum et al. 1993; Folstein et al. 1975), which assesses general cognitive functioning and is sensitive to detecting cognitive impairment secondary to delirium and dementia. Several other scales that directly assess decision-making capacity are commercially available (e.g., the MacArthur Competence Assessment Tool), and these have been validated in geriatric populations, research populations, and in the medically ill (Ganzini et al. 2004). To date, more than 30 capacity-assessment tools have been evaluated, and these instruments have been generally found to have high interrater reliability and validity and have been systematically reviewed and discussed elsewhere (Okai et al. 2007). There will of course be times when the patient lacks the capacity to give or withhold consent for treatment. In such situations, a surrogate decision-maker must be sought, although in emergencies, *beneficence* outweighs *autonomy*, and physicians can provide treatment. With regard to the surrogate decision-maker, state law or administrative codes as well as statutes may dictate a hierarchical, lineage-based flow of authority. Most commonly, the hierarchy is as follows: spouse, eldest adult child, parents, sibling, etc. As discussed in Chap. 4, disputes among these individuals may arise when their loved one is incapacitated, and in such cases, it is critical to help the family focus on what the patient would have wanted. In maintaining this focus, the psychiatric consultant will have to attend to the family systems theory issues discussed in Chap. 4.

Informed Consent

Informed consent is a process by which a patient agrees to a particular treatment after having understood its potential benefits, risks, and alternatives. Involving both the patient and the treatment team, this step is typically documented in writing in the medical record. No matter the length of the informed consent process—which generally parallels the complexity and the risks associated with the medical procedure in question—documentation of this process in the medical record is critical.

Involuntary Hospitalization

Sometimes a patient is unwilling to be psychiatrically hospitalized despite this being necessary for their well being, and in such cases they may be admitted without their consent. This process—involuntary hospitalization—subtends both medicolegal and ethical issues for the treatment team, the psychiatric consultant, and the patient. In general, involuntary hospitalization should be avoided except when absolutely necessary for the safety of the patient or of others or in circumstances when the patient cannot care for him or herself. To protect the patient's rights, statutory criteria for commitment exist, though they vary from state to state, and while only a court has the legal authority to involuntarily hospitalize a patient, psychiatrists (or licensed psychologists, depending on state laws) may *initiate* an involuntary hospitalization (for a specified period of time, e.g., 72 hours), a process which is often referred to, informally, as a "hold" or "petition," depending on the state and jurisdiction. Commonly the statutory criteria include: (1) the inability of the patient to care for himself; (2) evidence of imminent dangerousness to self or others, and (3) a reasonable expectation that the patient's condition is "treatable." We should note that the "inability to care for oneself" criterion does not apply in many states. Also, the "least restrictive" legal standard is often used to guard against unnecessary hospitalization. This is of particular importance in situations in which the patient might be treated in an outpatient setting or partial hospitalization setting.

6.4   Summary

Ethical and medicolegal issues are an inherent part of *difficult psychiatric consultations* and, as we have illustrated, create special challenges for the consulting psychiatrist working with both pediatric (Ascherman and Rubin 2008) and adult populations (Arras and Steinbock 1998; Gutheil et al. 2005). Among the key issues which must frequently be addressed are: *autonomy, nonmaleficence, beneficence,* and *justice*. Additionally, the consulting psychiatrist should be savvy regarding the state laws related to involuntary hospitalization as well as the process by which this occurs. Finally, it is critical for the consulting psychiatrist working with the difficult psychiatric consultation must have a strong working understanding of confidentiality, privilege, and the related limitations of these aspects of treatment/consultation.

References

American Academy of Child and Adolescent Psychiatry (2009) Code of ethics. American Academy of Child and Adolescent Psychiatry, Washington, DC

American Psychiatric Association (2009) American psychiatric association: the principles of medical ethics with special annotations especially applicable to psychiatry. American Psychiatric Association, Arlington, VA

Appelbaum PS (2007) Clinical practice. Assessment of patients' competence to consent to treatment. N Engl J Med 357(18):1834–1840

Appelbaum PS, Grisso T (1988) Assessing patients' capacities to consent to treatment. N Engl J Med 319(25):1635–1638

Arras JD, Steinbock B (1998) Ethical issues in modern medicine, 5th edn. Mayfield, Mountain View, CA

Ascherman LI, Rubin S (2008) Current ethical issues in child and adolescent psychiatry. Child Adolesc Psychiatr Clin N Am 17:21–35

U.S. Congress, House of Representatives, Committee of Conference (1996) Health Insurance Portability and Accountability Act of 1996, 31 July 1996

Crum RM, Anthony JC, Bassett SS et al (1993) Population-based norms for the Mini-Mental State examination by age and educational level. JAMA 269(18):2386–2391

Edelstein L (1967) The Hippocratic Oath: text, translation and interpretation. In: Temkin O, Temkin CL (eds) Ancient medicine: selected papers of Ludwig Edelstein. Johns Hopkins Press, Baltimore, MD, pp 3–64

Folstein MF, Folstein SE, McHugh PR (1975) "Mini-mental state" a practical method for grading the cognitive state of patients for the clinician. J Psychiatr Res 12(3):189–198

Ganzini L, Volicer L, Nelson WA et al (2004) Ten myths about decision making capacity. J Am Med Dir Assoc 5(4):263–267

Gutheil TG, Simon RI, Hilliard JT (2005) The wrong handle: flawed fixes of medicolegal problems in psychiatry and the law. J Am Acad Psychiatry Law 33(4):432–436

Levenson JL (2013) Legal issues in the interface of medicine and psychiatry. http://www.primarypsychiatry.com/aspx/articledetail.aspx?articleid=117. Accessed 1 Feb 2013

Mahajan AP, Sayles JN, Patel VA et al (2008) Stigma in the HIV/AIDS epidemic: a review of the literature and recommendations for the way forward. AIDS 22(Suppl 2):S67–S79

Majumdar SK (1995) Ethical aspects of the Hippocratic Oath and its relevance to contemporary medicine. Bull Ind Inst Hist Med Hyderabad 25(1–2):150–169

Okai D, Owen G, McGuire H et al (2007) Mental capacity in psychiatric patients: systematic review. Br J Psychiatry 191:291–297

Pantilat SZ, Lo B (2005) Ethical issues in the hospitalized patient. In: Wachter RM, Lee G, Harry H (eds) Hospital medicine, 2nd edn. Lippincott Williams & Wilkins, New York, NY, pp 119–128

Schetky DH (2007) Ethics. In: Andrés M, Volkmar FR (eds) Lewis's child and adolescent psychiatry: a comprehensive textbook, 4th edn. Lippincott Williams & Wilkins, Philadelphia, PA, pp 17–22

Simon RI, Schindler BA, Levenson JL (2005) Legal issues. In: Levenson JL (ed) The American psychiatric publishing textbook of psychosomatic medicine. American Psychiatric Publishing, Washington, DC, pp 37–54

Swanepoel M (2009) The development of the interface between law, medicine and psychiatry: medico-legal perspectives in history. Potchefstroom Electr Law J 12(4):124–360

Wecht CH (2005) The history of legal medicine. J Am Acad Psychiatry Law 33(2):245–251

The Culture 7

*I look to a day when people will not be judged by the color of
their skin, but by the content of their character*
—Martin Luther King Jr. (1929–1968)

Up to this point we have emphasized the importance of bringing clarity to difficult
clinical consultations by understanding the vulnerabilities and integrating the
strengths of the patient, the family system, and the treatment team. In this chapter
we will focus on how cultural competence may facilitate communication, diagnosis, and treatment in patient care. To grasp the varying personalities within a group
that is part of the larger shared system, it is necessary to consider an overarching,
unifying system that influences all of its members—culture.

7.1 A Working Definition of Culture

For our purposes, we define *culture* as the amalgam of languages, social customs,
traditions, beliefs, and values shared by a group of people linked by family, race,
ethnicity, region, or culture of origin. The USA is home to many different cultures,
races, and ethnicities, and this diversity has enriched the nation in a number of
areas: science, literature, the arts, politics, sports, and religion. Not a static concept,
culture can change over time as people acclimate to a new environment and later
begin to influence it. For example, when immigrants arrive in the USA, they may
initially hold on to their country's cultural traditions, though over time many
incorporate the traditions of their adopted country. Examples of this are seen with
immigrants from Ireland or Mexico, who gradually adapted to the social norms of
the USA without letting go of rituals like the annual celebration of Saint Patrick's
Day or Cinco de Mayo, which are widely recognized as symbols of how Irish and
Hispanics have contributed to US culture. Acclimation can also apply to "small
world" situations, such as when a family moves from one state or region (e.g., the
South) or neighborhood (e.g., the West Side) to another that has a different set of
beliefs and values. In Fig. 7.1 we see what is referred to as the culture iceberg, a

S.V. Delgado and J.R. Strawn, *Difficult Psychiatric Consultations*,
DOI 10.1007/978-3-642-39552-9_7, © Springer-Verlag Berlin Heidelberg 2014

"Surface" Aspects of Culture

Skin color
Food choices
Customs
Music
Language

**"Deep" Aspects of Culture
(not observable)**

Attitudes toward life
Social values
Religion and moral values
Family rituals
Beliefs in health and medicine
Non-verbal behaviors, social etiquette

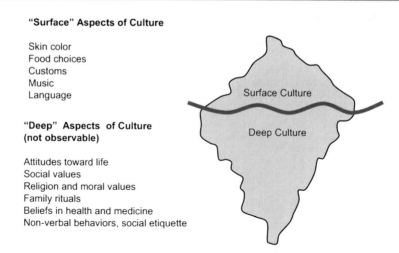

Fig. 7.1 Culture may be understood in terms of two distinct levels. Surface aspects of culture are often apparent during cursory interactions, while deep aspects of culture are often not observable and, in many circumstances, are of critical importance in working with the difficult psychiatric consultation

visual representation of both surface and deep cultural factors. Frequently, individuals base their impressions of a given culture on surface factors (e.g., color of skin, the accent from native language, or social etiquette). This is stereotyping, which, needless to say, involves lack of appreciation of deep cultural aspects that are more representative of true beliefs and values. An example of mutual stereotyping is as follows: A psychiatry resident in psychotherapy supervision is disappointed upon meeting her supervisor, Dr. Cortez, as she had hoped he would be Hispanic and could help her with two Mexican patients she has started seeing. When she states, "It's ok if you are not Hispanic. Many people with Hispanic names are white, have been raised in the US, and aren't true Hispanics," the supervisor is surprised, as he assumes that his name is enough to indicate his Hispanic descent. When he asks what has led the resident to think that he is not "a true Hispanic," she replies, "You don't look Hispanic, and you don't have an accent." Though the faculty physician is initially shocked, he uses this interaction as a teachable moment and helps the resident openly discuss cultural issues and how they might affect her psychotherapeutic work with Hispanic patients. This example captures how easily stereotyping can occur. The faculty physician has expectations that the resident will somehow know his name represents his cultural heritage and stereotypes her as not being culturally sensitive. The resident stereotypes the faculty physician, who does not look or speak "like a Hispanic." This interaction shows how biases involving surface cultural factors can result in misleading, even hurtful, assumptions.

Cross (1988) has advanced the widely accepted definition of cultural competence as "a set of congruent behaviors, attitudes, and policies that come together in a system, agency, or among professionals, and enable that system, agency, or those professionals to work effectively in cross-cultural situations."

Level of Cultural Competence Necessary for Treatment Teams

- Understanding that diversity is more than differences of race and ethnicity
- Ability to assess cultural realities for the patient and family
- Respect for and willingness to learn the cultural specificity for the patient and family
- Allowing for multicultural members in the treatment teams
- In children, learning about culturally specific toys, games, and videos
- Availability of interpreters (essential)

7.2   Culture Shock

When a person moves from a stable culture to one that is unfamiliar to them, they may experience what is colloquially termed *culture shock*. Ticho (1971) described culture shock as a result of a sudden change from an "average expectable environment to a strange and unpredictable one." The complex process that follows such a disruption undoubtedly will have psychological repercussions. The intensity, form, and content of the psychological changes are unique to each person, based on the cognitive and affective flexibility, temperament, and attachment style that was present before moving to a new cultural environment. *Culture shock* is masterfully described in Garza-Guerrero's (1974) classic psychoanalytic paper, in which he defines the phenomenon as "a reactive process stemming from the impact of a new culture upon those who attempt to merge with it as a newcomer." Garza-Guerrero adds that culture shock profoundly tests the adequacy of an individual's personality functioning, as there will be an initial phase of mourning the abandoned culture that severely threatens identity. Further stating that "three definable elements invariably constitute common denominators of this phenomenon," Garza-Guerrero discusses the psychological challenges a person goes through when changing cultural environments (Table 7.1). He proposes that a mourning process is a prerequisite to working through the healthy inhibitory forces seen in adhering to customs and traditions of the past culture and in the resistance to those of the new one. When the mourning process occurs, it allows for the assimilation of the new culture's values and beliefs in a mature manner, providing a healthy resolution of the culture shock, which is viewed by Ticho, as a self-limiting crisis (1971).

It is hardly a surprise that culture shock is a stressful, anxiety-provoking situation, a violent encounter that puts the newcomer's coping mechanisms to the test, challenging the stability of his or her psychic organization. When this crisis is resolved, emotional growth may emerge; if it is not resolved successfully, diverse

Table 7.1 Culture shock challenges (Garza-Guerrero 1974)

Phase 1	Phase 2	Phase 3
Cultural encounter	Reorganization	New sense of self
Identity crisis	*Mourning process*	*Reshaping of self and others*
Exploring differences and similarities	Gradual acceptance	New ego identity with less fear of integrating both cultural worlds in self
Mourning identity as part of a group	Working through mourning of ideal self	Continual reediting process of self
Exaggerated idealization of original culture	A more realistic view of new culture	Accepting that the longing for original culture will remain
Exaggerated importance to loss of friends and family	Attempt to merge by creating new friends	Feeling of belonging to new group
Social inhibition in new culture	Selective identifications with new culture	Social acceptance of self and others

degrees of stagnation and even pathological regression may occur—brought on by the profound loss of a variety of love and transitional objects in the abandoned culture. Among others, these losses are family, friends, language, music, food, and culturally determined values, customs, and attitudes.

Most academic hospitals have specialty programs that attract patients from across the country and, at times, the globe. In many of these cases, if not all, the patient and family leave their original culture under duress after the diagnosis of a difficult-to-treat illness, and if the move happens abruptly due to medical necessity (treatment of burns, bone marrow transplants, atypical gastrointestinal surgeries, etc.), the intensity of the situation may contribute to an acute stress reaction, not to be confused with severe psychopathology.

When the psychiatric consultation requested by the treatment team includes an element relating to cultural issues, it is necessary for the consultant to be culturally sensitive. Table 7.1 can help identify the phase in which the patient and family find themselves, and in using this chart, the consultant can tailor the interventions needed to improve the treatment outcomes. It will be quite different for a family if a member becomes ill during the identity crisis phase, which may result in the patient displaying social inhibition with the treatment team. On the other hand, if the family member becomes ill during reshaping-of-self-and-others phase, the psychiatric consultant may not be needed, as the family system will have gone through the mourning necessary to allow for a mature and healthy way of addressing adversity and will have a social support group in their current environment.

As described in Chaps. 2 and 3, when an individual has a difficult temperament, limited cognitive functioning, and an insecure attachment style, they will have more pronounced problems in changing environments and can regress in a pathological manner to the point of requiring urgent psychiatric care. In such situations, the psychiatric consultant can facilitate interventions by the treatment team, suggesting concrete actions that may help patients feel less alone in a different cultural environment. The team should be encouraged to request help from a culturally sensitive social work staff and to provide patients with the time and means for communication (by phone or electronic media) with family or friends, both near and in other countries. By learning about the treatments commonly provided for a patient's condition in their original culture, the treatment team can carefully compare them with the current recommendations, and discussing with the patient and family what led to the differences in medical approaches. Furthermore, acknowledging the difficulties with the transition they have experienced can significantly reduce the impact of the culture shock.

Cultural Sensitivity and Cultural Competence

Cultural sensitivity involves members of a medical treatment team making an effort to recognize that biases (either conscious or unconscious) regarding diverse populations may influence their approach to the best-practice patient care as well as the way they communicate with culturally different patients and families. Some team members may be more adept at recognizing and understanding that certain patients fear making eye contact, while others prefer that family members speak for them. Still others bring their young children or all of their family to the bedside. When these culture-specific behaviors are openly discussed and the treatment team understands the reasons for them, a rapport is established that strengthens the alliance of everyone supporting the patient, encourages his or her compliance with treatment, and improves medical outcomes (Lie et al. 2008; Qureshi et al. 2008).

Old-School Values

Sometimes a cultural dilemma arises from a regional or generational issue. We use the term *old-school values* to refer to a philosophy whereby long-held values and traditions are shared by the family system and community. These are typically based on religious beliefs. At times old-school values may result in a patient's or family's unwillingness to consider evidence-based treatment approaches. This most commonly occurs when grandparents or elder family members participate in the best-practice treatment planning for a patient, but it is not limited to that demographic. Younger members of a family that is loyal to traditional or cultural values and beliefs may also refuse treatment interventions. Many believe that medications are being overused and are dangerous and use the medication warnings to support their reluctance. In consultation psychiatry, the term *old-school values* refers to the perception that modern medicine promotes pharmacological solutions and stands in opposition to traditional, core beliefs. Situations that involve these perceptions need to be approached with sensitivity. The psychiatric consultant might suggest that the treatment team take a down-to-earth approach and allow ample time to explain the risks in not pursuing treatment. When team members rush through their recommendations, it is, in essence, not being culturally sensitive. Many families are used to taking time to talk with one other and value the extended face-to-face encounter. To address this issue, some urban hospitals have initiated culturally sensitive patient groups and family support groups as part of the patient-centered care mission, which has improved the sense of partnership between individual patients, families, and their treatment teams. The groups allow patients and families to speak about old-school values, and many are surprised to find people in general share their struggles, no matter their regional or cultural disparities.

Socioeconomic Aspects of Culture

The cultural challenges and obstacles a psychiatric consultant can face are not limited to race and ethnicity, as differences can also occur at the socioeconomic level. It is likely that members of a treatment team and the consultant have encountered conflict when providing help to those of different socioeconomic status—whether the patient is part of an indigent population or an affluent one. A person or family with low income may agree with the treatment team's recommendations while failing to mention (out of shame or guilt) that the recommendations are unrealistic for them because they lack the financial resources to carry them out. The result is a noncompliance issue (Grupp-Phelan et al. 2007).

The Well-Intentioned Physician Thrown a Cultural Curve

Early in his residency, a physician volunteers in a midwestern rural community and recruits a diverse group of residents from several specialty programs to provide medical services. The physician is particularly interested in preventive medicine and gives a brief presentation to a group of families about the importance of vegetables and fruits in their diet. He brings bags of apples to distribute, and as he passes them out, he feels embarrassed as several people began to giggle and talk to each other. He stops the presentation, feeling he has done something terribly wrong. A spokesperson for the group gives him a big smile and points to her missing teeth, stating, "We can't eat apples." Clearly, this community has suffered from poverty for years, and many adults had poor dental care, which made the choice of apples unwise. The families were kind enough to share that they appreciated the visit and jokingly added, "Bring apple sauce next time." He did!

Patients or families of higher socioeconomic status may demand treatment from individuals of organizational importance (e.g., the division director or senior physician within the department). Surely the reader will recognize a familiar anxiety-provoking question from many such patients: "Who's your supervisor?" In asking this question, or in demanding treatment from more senior physicians, these patients and families may be conveying the perception that they have received *second-class treatment* and that they or their family members have not been appropriately examined and diagnosed because they have not been seen by the most experienced physician. Like many people of varying income or status, they may fear accepting the seriousness of the medical or psychiatric illness, but culturally it may be difficult for them to acknowledge that though they have financial advantages, money cannot provide the optimistic outcome they hope for. The treatment of patients from affluent backgrounds and of those from lower socioeconomic circumstances received attention in the psychotherapy literature (Mckamy 1976; Stone 1972). In this literature, an important distinction is made: whereas the outpatient "chooses" to be a part of their treatment, the inpatient with an acute medical or psychiatric illness—regardless of socioeconomic circumstances— often does not have the luxury of choosing to be a patient. Moreover, the literature concerning socioeconomic status and clinical treatment suggests that treatment team members "change care based on their patients' SES... [and that] these changes may contribute to measured socioeconomic disparities in health care" (Bernheim et al. 2008).

The Entitled, Affluent Patient

Mr. Baker, a 38-year-old, somewhat timid executive, is admitted to the epilepsy-monitoring unit of a large, urban, academic medical center for worsening of his partial complex seizures. During the hospitalization, he is initially treated with divalproex (current level 90 ug/mL) by the inpatient neurology team, but nevertheless continues to have daily seizures. Both Mr. Baker and his partner are concerned that he is not receiving "name brand" Depakote® (divalproex) in the hospital and believe this explains his continued seizing. The patient's partner, during morning bedside rounds, yells at the neurology treatment team for providing "inferior care." The team requests a psychiatric consultation, as they feel the patient and his partner are being "difficult to work with." The consulting psychiatrist meets with the patient that afternoon and plans to meet with the neurology treatment team, the patient, and his partner—a 40-year-old executive at a large multinational corporation—later that day to discuss additional treatment options. However, the treatment team is urgently called to evaluate a patient in the neuro-intensive care unit in status epilepticus and is late to the planned meeting with Mr. Baker and his partner. As they approach the meeting room, the consulting psychiatrist observes that both Mr. Baker and his partner are angry at the treatment team, and upon their arrival, Mr. Baker's partner, pointing to his watch, exclaims, "You're 25 min late. I had to cancel an important meeting to be here." In an accusing tone, he then interrupts the attending neurologist, saying, "We could have chosen to go to a more renowned medical center..." The psychiatric consultant intervenes and apologizes for their wait (Joining, Chap. 4), adding, "I'm worried that even if we did help you transfer to a more renowned treatment center, you might still feel helpless and afraid for your partner." Surprisingly, the patient and his partner were able to talk about their sense of helplessness, admitting, "We don't know what to do. We're not used to feeling helpless. We usually get what we want. When will the seizures stop?" It's important to note, however, that when events do not evolve as well as in the above example, the consultant will benefit from assessing whether the patient or family has had changes in observed temperament, cognitive and affective flexibility, and attachment style (see Chaps. 2 and 3) and design an intervention that is sensitive to their level of functioning.

In this difficult psychiatric consultation, we see the pertinence of cultural sensitivity from several vantages. The psychiatric consultant was keenly aware that the patient and his partner may have elicited countertransference reactions on the part of the treatment team, whether related to their being gay or to their affluence (Chap. 2). First, regarding the issue of homosexuality, and despite recent shifts toward tolerance and acceptance, some treatment team members may experience unconscious discomfort in working with same-sex partners because of their religious or cultural beliefs (Smith and Mathews 2007). These individuals may spend less time with the patient, may be less able to listen to the patient, and may struggle to engage with the patient and his or her partner. In being attentive to these issues, the psychiatric consultant becomes a cultural interpreter. Second, regarding the patient's affluence, some team members may experience unconscious discomfort in working with wealthy patients. Specifically, these team members may struggle with feelings of envy or anger, may feel intimidated, and, in some cases, acquiesce to the patient's demands, which might be at odds with the patient's best interests (McKamy 1976). These issues may be accentuated in pediatric consultations, as the illness of a child is difficult for any parent to accept, and some with substantial financial resources may believe they can "purchase" the best treatment and in doing so alleviate their child's pain and suffering (Stone 1972).

7.3   Mental Health Across Cultures

The concept of mental health varies across cultures, though there is a shared understanding that those with good mental health have the capacity to forge and sustain loving and stable relationships, to work productively, and to enjoy leisure pursuits. According to the World Health Organization (2011), "mental health is not just the absence of mental disorder. It is defined as a state of well-being in which every individual realizes his or her own potential, can cope with the normal stresses of life, can work productively and fruitfully, and is able to make a contribution to his or her community." A person's culture will influence what is considered "the norm" for loving and stable relationships. In the USA, for example, some parents are expected to send their children away when they enter college, so the children "leaving the nest" can create independent adult lives, while in other cultures such a separation is considered uncaring to the parents and a sign of family conflict. Because actions and behaviors can be perceived differently by those of other cultures, the treatment team should consider the patient's culture and allow this to influence the type of assessment, diagnosis, and best-practice treatment plan they formulate, as well as the role their family will have in the patient's care. It is essential for the psychiatric consultant to have some understanding of the patient's culture and to help the treatment team recognize the impact it may have on the clinical presentation of his or her medical or psychiatric illness (Fung et al 2008). Patients and families from certain cultures may view medical and psychiatric treatment with mistrust and, due to culture issues, may not share the severity of the symptoms out of fear of treatment. This is particularly relevant for some Hispanic and Asian cultures, in which close-knit family networks are common and younger members rely on elders' wisdom when decisions need to be made. Many African Americans may rely on a network that is not limited to family and friends but includes their clergy and fellow churchgoers. Dana states that members of this group "feel more comfortable with support services found in churches...than with formal mental health services" (Dana 2002; Davey and Watson 2008; Gara et al. 2012).

Cultural sensitivity is particularly important in working with cases involving mental illness. Members of racial minority groups may delay seeking mental health services when they have a negative view of mental illness or fear being stigmatized. This can lead certain populations to seek mental health services when they are in an acute phase of the psychiatric illness, which can result in an increase of involuntary hospitalization and consequently reinforce a negative view of mental health providers. It is unfortunate that some family members, due cultural issues, may delay the evaluation of their loved one, thereby prolonging the suffering and severity of illness. Patients and families from different cultures often perceive the use of medication as a sign of weakness and believe taking "mind-altering agents" involves a loss of control and/or loss of self. Thus, issues of compliance are a significant problem for patients in some cultures.

Interventions to Address Cultural Factors That May Interfere with Treatment

In Table 7.2 we review the many treatment barriers that stem from the cultural situations described above and provide practical interventions for the psychiatric consultant to consider when providing help to treatment teams.

The use of this table allows the psychiatric consultant to provide practical interventions for the treatment team to consider when providing help to patient and families while receiving care in a medical setting or after discharge.

7.4   Working with Interpreters

If a patient speaks a different language than the treatment team or psychiatric consultant, interpreters should be utilized. We have occasionally observed that in such situations, some team members inadvertently relied on children or other family members to interpret. However, the family may be more attuned and anxious about the patient's illness or pain, and these concerns may influence the translation.

The use of well-trained and culturally sensitive interpreters can help establish a working alliance with patients and their families and facilitate treatment compliance. In recent years, at large and small medical centers alike, interpretation has

Table 7.2 Cultural factors that may interfere with treatment

Treatment barriers	Culture	Interventions by psychiatric consultant
Culture-based fear of medical providers/ medications Stigma and myths	Country Regional Old-school values	• Suggest in-house support groups • Offer reading materials in patient's native language • Provide examples of expected outcomes • Increase length of interactions at bedside
Use of herbal or alternative medicine Religious traditions	Rituals Spiritual factors Religion	• Consult with holistic medicine practitioner • Consult with chaplain or pastor • Facilitate access to family's church leaders • Allow for local healers, with limits
Dietary problems	Limited access to native foods	• Provide information about local grocery stores with native foods
Socioeconomic factors	Limited financial resources	• Financial counseling from hospital • Financial support from patient services • Help with transportation
Limited availability of services	Rural communities Limited financial support Limited insurance coverage	• Direct call from team to local social services • Teach family to provide medical care after discharge, when appropriate • Hospital financial and patient services facilitate access to local services
Racial and ethnic minorities	Different countries of origin Racial issues Gay, lesbian, bisexual, and transgender	• Call local community groups of similar minority • Reassure care is not biased by sharing examples of other patients • Dialogue with office of diversity and inclusion of similar race team members
Legal issues	Immigration	• Discuss with patient and family openly • Consult legal services

been facilitated though the use of "phone in" services as well as interpreters who are physically present, which has greatly helped the decision-making role of patients in partnership with their providers. However, there are some limitations to the use of interpreters. First, because the interpreter may miss or may be unable to communicate affective elements of the encounter, it is critical for the treatment team or consultant to maintain rapport and eye contact with the patient and family during the exchange. The consultant or team members should use the first-person form of address, should face the patient, and direct questions and comments to him or her, not to the interpreter. The interpreter may occasionally pause to ask for an explanation or clarification of terms, and the treatment team will need to exercise patience and trust that the interpreter will convey all that is said in the presence of all individuals, including things spoken as asides. When possible, it is helpful for the treatment team or psychiatric consultant to meet with the interpreter both before the encounter (to discuss the approach to the patient) and after (to discuss the degree to which there may have been impairment in communication). Interpreting language alone is not enough to facilitate communication or to understand the patient and family. The cultural context surrounding the illness and diagnosis may not be readily apparent. Specifically, the anxiety or sadness with which a patient responds to a particular diagnosis or intervention may diverge from the consultant or treatment team's expected reaction based on their culture of reference. Also, literal interpretations sometimes hinder communication; it is important that interpreters retain the "flavor" of the original interpretation. For the treatment team, inadequate communication may (1) impact the development of a therapeutic relationship and (2) impair understanding of the cultural context of the patient's behavior.

7.5 Culture in *DSM-IV-TR* and *DSM-5*

The World Health Organization (WHO 2011) suggests that the clinical picture of a psychiatric illness presents similarly regardless of cultural factors. Nevertheless, the way a person or family recognizes the signs of a mental illness is strongly influenced by their culture. The *Diagnostic and Statistical Manual of Mental Disorders, 4th Edition, Text Revision (DSM-IV-TR* 2000), Appendix I, provides an outline for cultural formulation divided into two sections. The first section is designed to supplement the multiaxial diagnostic assessment to assist the clinician in systematically evaluating and reporting the impact of the individual's cultural context as relevant to clinical care:

DSM-IV-TR Outline for Cultural Formulation
• Cultural identity of the individual
• Cultural explanations of the individual's illness
• Cultural factors related to psychosocial environment and levels of functioning
• Cultural elements of the relationship between the individual and the clinician
• Overall cultural assessment for diagnosis and care

The second section is a glossary of culture-bound syndromes, a combination of psychiatric and somatic symptoms that are considered to be a recognizable disease only within a specific society or culture (*DSM-IV-TR* 200, Table 7.3). In *Diagnostic and Statistical Manual of Mental Disorders, 5th Edition (DSM-5)*, the culture-bound construct is replaced by three concepts: cultural syndrome, culture idiom of distress, and cultural experience or perceived cause. These concepts can be elicited during the clinical encounter. Further, in *DSM-5*, this section was expanded to include a semistructured cultural formulation interview (CFI), a set of 16 questions which allow providers to better understand the impact of culture on the patient's clinical presentation. This approach allows clinicians to better understand "values, orientation, knowledge, and practices that individuals derive from membership in diverse group" (*DSM-5* 2013) and focuses on a myriad of domains:

Table 7.3 Selected culture-bound syndromes in *DSM-IV* and *DSM-5*

Name	Geography/culture	Description
Ataque de nervios	Latinos	• Episode of uncontrollable yelling, tearfulness, tremulousness, and somatic symptos which may be accompanied by aggression • May be accompanied by dissociation, seizure-like/fainting episodes, and suicidal ideation • Individuals may have a sense of "losing control" • Precipitants may include stress within the family • *Clinicians should consider the possibility of the following DSM-5 disorders: Panic disorder, dissociative disorder, conversion disorder, and unspecified anxiety disorder*
Koro	China, Malaysia, Asia	• Episodic, acute-onset, severe anxiety and fears that the genitalia have retracted into the body • May occur in groups of individuals • *Clinicians should consider the possibility of the following DSM-5 disorders: Panic disorder, conversion disorder, delusional disorder, and unspecified anxiety disorder*
Mal de Ojo	Mediterranean cultures and Hispanic	• Literally translated as "evil eye" • An episode of restlessness, crying and somatic symptoms including diarrhea, vomiting, and fever which may be more common in young children, but can occur in adults • *Clinicians should consider the possibility of the following DSM-5 disorders: Panic disorder, dissociative disorder, conversion disorder, and unspecified anxiety disorder*
zār	Ethiopia, Somalia, Egypt, Sudan, Iran, and other North African and Middle Eastern Societies	• Afflicted individuals believe that a spirit may have possessed the individual • Accompanied by dissociation and during the episode, individuals may yell, laugh uncontrollably, sing, cry, or become physically aggressive. Additionally, the individual may note withdrawal, may refuse to participate in activities of daily living, and in some circumstances, may "develop a long-term relationship with the possessing spirit"

Selected Aspects of the *DSM-5* Cultural Formulation Interview (CFI)
- Cultural definition of the problem
- Cultural perceptions of cause, context, and support
- Role of cultural identity
- Cultural factors affecting current help seeking
- Cultural context of the clinician–patient relationship

Additionally, the CFI may facilitate understanding regarding the overlap of culturally "distinctive symptoms and diagnostic criteria" as well as "difficulty in diagnostic assessment owing to significant differences in the cultural, religious, or socioeconomic backgrounds of the clinician and the individual" (*DSM-5* 2013). For additional information regarding the incorporation of the cultural elements from *DSM* in the clinical encounter and its influence on diagnostic formulations, we refer the reader to the following thorough reviews: Dinh et al. (2012), Harris et al. (2008), Lu (2006) and Mezzich et al. (1999).

7.6 Summary

Culture is the ever-present factor that influences the ways we communicate with patients, inhibits or enhances our understanding of their illnesses, and provides the context that explains their reactions to the event. The context may be the culture of the family, the culture of the treatment team's hospital, and/or the culture that defines the legal standards in patient care. Bringing clarity to difficult psychiatric consultations often requires a culturally-informed understanding of the vulnerabilities and strengths of the patient, the family system, and the treatment team, will. In this chapter we have focused on how cultural competence may facilitate communication, diagnosis, and treatment.

References

American Psychiatric Association (2000) Diagnostic and statistical manual of mental disorders: DSM-IV-TR, 4th edn. American Psychiatric Association, Washington, DC, text rev

American Psychiatric Association (2013) Diagnostic and statistical manual of mental disorders: DSM-5, 5th edn. American Psychiatric Association, Washington, DC, pp 750–751

Bernheim SM, Ross JS, Krumholz HM et al (2008) Influence of patients' socioeconomic status on clinical management decisions: a qualitative study. Ann Fam Med 6(1):53–59

Cross TL (1988) Service to minority populations: cultural competence continuum. Focal Point 3:1–4

Dana RH (2002) Mental health services for African Americans: a cultural/racial perspective. Cult Divers Ethn Minor Psychol 8:3–18

Davey MP, Watson MF (2008) Engaging African Americans in therapy: integrating a public policy and family therapy perspective. Contemp Fam Ther 30:31–47

Dinh NM, Groleau D, Kirmayer LJ et al (2012) Influence of the DSM-IV outline for cultural formulation on multidisciplinary case conferences in mental health. Anthropol Med 19 (3):261–276

Fung K, Andermann L, Zaretsky A et al (2008) An integrative approach to cultural competence in the psychiatric curriculum. Acad Psychiatry 32:272–282

Gara MA, Vega WA, Arndt S et al (2012) Influence of patient race and ethnicity on clinical assessment in patients with affective disorders. Arch Gen Psychiatry 69(6):593–600

Garza-Guerrero AC (1974) Culture shock: its mourning and the vicissitudes of identity. J Am Psychoanal Ass 22:408–429

Grupp-Phelan J, Delgado SV, Kelleher KJ (2007) Failure of psychiatric referrals from the pediatric emergency department. BMC Emerg Med 7:12

Harris TL, McQuery J, Raab B (2008) Multicultural psychiatric education: using the DSM-IV-TR outline for cultural formulation to improve resident cultural competence. Acad Psychiatry 32:306–312

Lie DA, Boker J, Crandall S et al (2008) Revising the tool for assessing cultural competence training (TACCT) for curriculum evaluation: findings derived from seven US schools and expert consensus. Med Educ Online 13, 1–11. Available at: http://www.pubmedcentral.nih.gov/articlerender.fcgi?artid=2743012&tool=pmcentrez&rendertype=abstract

Lu FG (2006) DSM-IV outline for cultural formulation: bringing culture into the clinical encounter. Focus 4:9–10

McKamy EH (1976) Social work with the wealthy. Soc Casework 57:254–258

Mezzich JE, Kirmayer LJ, Kleinman A et al (1999) The place of culture in DSM-IV. J Nerv Ment Dis 187(8):457–464

Qureshi A, Collazos F, Ramos M, Casas M et al (2008) Cultural competency training in psychiatry. Eur Psychiatry 23(1):49–58

Smith DM, Mathews WC (2007) Physicians' attitudes toward homosexuality and HIV: survey of a California Medical Society- revisited (PATHH-II). J Homosex 52(3–4):1–9

Stone MH (1972) Treating the wealthy and their children. J Child Psychother 1:15–46

Ticho G (1971) Cultural aspects of transference and countertransference. Bull Menninger Clin 35:313–334

World Health Organization. Mental health (2011). http://www.who.int/topics/mental_health/en/

The Clinical Presentation

8

Make everything as simple as possible, but not simpler
—Albert Einstein (1879–1955)

Presenting case material to colleagues requires preparation, whether the presentation is to be made casually during bedside rounds or in the formal environment of a national meeting. It is rewarding when a presentation is well received, particularly because it may prove helpful to other clinicians, allied health professionals, and researchers. Regardless of the setting, the presenter's goal is to share their knowledge based on observations they have made and lessons they have learned from the case or cases. The most time-consuming aspect of the presentation is collecting and organizing as much information as possible about the patients, their families, and others who were involved in the patients' care. Once these tasks are complete, the presenter must summarize the information and place it within the context of treatment data and consensus approaches. Tailoring the talk to the audience is also of paramount importance. Different groups will invariably come from different disciplines, and the presentation will need to be tailored to accommodate each audience's background, interests and goals.

8.1 Presentations

There are a multitude of presentation formats for sharing and discussing clinical cases, diagnostic formulations or dilemmas, treatment approaches, and ethical issues. These presentation formats vary in terms of the number and type of participants, the use of multimedia, the availability of continuing medical education credits, etc. (Hull et al. 1989). Below, we describe the most common formats for clinical presentations and the challenges and unique features of each, though we recognize that aspects of these presentations will vary by organization, institution, and region.

S.V. Delgado and J.R. Strawn, *Difficult Psychiatric Consultations*,
DOI 10.1007/978-3-642-39552-9_8, © Springer-Verlag Berlin Heidelberg 2014

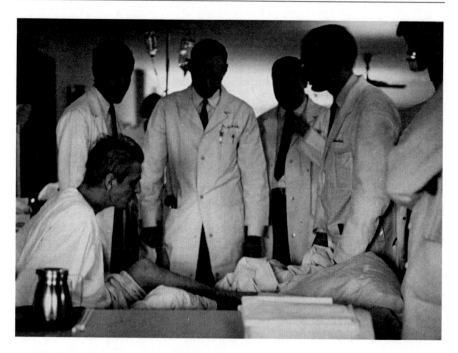

Fig. 8.1 Bedside teaching rounds c. 1960 Photo by Roy Perry. National Library of Medicine

Teaching Rounds Presentations

Teaching rounds have been the tradition in academic hospitals in which faculty members work closely with trainees, typically on a daily basis, so as to educate them about clinical approaches for patient care (Fig. 8.1). Faculty also use this model to teach trainees to present cases with specific complex issues in a succinct, effective, and collegial manner. Generally, teaching rounds involve small groups of clinicians within a department and are usually scheduled daily to weekly, depending on the institution or department. Various members of the department may attend, including faculty, residents, interns, and nurses. In this context, the presenter can assume that most of those attending have a similar fund of knowledge regarding medical and psychiatric illnesses, and therefore the intent of the presentation is to highlight unique and unusual aspects of a particular patient, facilitating the discussion of new diagnostic, clinical, or treatment concepts. In these rounds, the presenter typically reviews the patient's history and the course of his or her medical or psychiatric illness, as well as diagnostic formulations and best-practice treatment plans. The presenter may find it helpful to utilize the table-based approach, as we have done throughout this book, to systematically integrate aspects of temperament, cognition, defense mechanisms, family systems, and ethical issues.

Clinical Case Conference Presentations

This type of conference permits clinicians to present material regarding complex cases and involves active discussion by participants about clinical formulations, diagnostic challenges, and/or best-practice treatment issues. A clinical case conference frequently utilizes an external discussant/moderator who approaches the case from one or two theoretical vantages. The discussant will also summarize the clinical material presented and may reformulate the material and expound on complex diagnostic or treatment issues. Importantly, the discussant is often charged with facilitating the discussion between the presenters and the audience members.

Grand Rounds Presentations

Historically, in teaching hospitals over the last century, "grand rounds" consisted of a regular gathering of students, resident physicians, attending physicians, and senior physicians who observed as a junior and senior colleague examined a patient (Fig. 8.2), then engaged in a "Socratic dialogue, that often led the audience in a step-by-step deciphering of the ailment" (Altman 2006). Over the last several decades, grand rounds have taken the form of didactic lectures (Altman 2006) that focus on epidemiologic findings, pathophysiology and risk factors for a given condition, and treatment approaches that rely on evidence-based medicine (Sackett et al. 1996). Modern grand rounds may still include the review of a case history, which allows a senior presenter to share the popular "clinical pearls" (Lorin et al. 2008). Despite its transformation over the recent years (from patient to participant focus), grand rounds remain a crucial element of medical education in, as Lawrence Altman, M.D. laments, "an era of proliferating subspecialties." Altman also notes that grand rounds serve myriad purposes, in that it "emphasizes a core body of knowledge that all physicians need to share and to keep abreast of. And the meetings serve a social function. With coffee cups and bagels or pizza in hand, doctors mingle with colleagues before and after grand rounds. For some, it is the only time they see one another during the week" (2006).

The grand rounds presenter should keep in mind that audience members will have varying levels of training and experience and may have different theoretical orientations with different expectations about how the clinical material is understood. It is unrealistic to expect that an experienced and knowledgeable clinician will always be a good speaker, or that a good speaker will be able to please all members of the audience. Nonetheless, it is imperative to provide one's clinical opinions with the best intentions, reminding the audience that the presentation is the synthesis of a great deal of information that the presenter believes is relevant, helpful, and current. It is important both to convey the material in a manner that is sensitive to the unique needs and perspectives of the audience (e.g., community-based physicians, subspecialty physicians, research faculty, advance practice nurses, psychologists, etc.) and to consider how the material will be viewed by the different disciplines present. The presenter should keep in mind the diverse

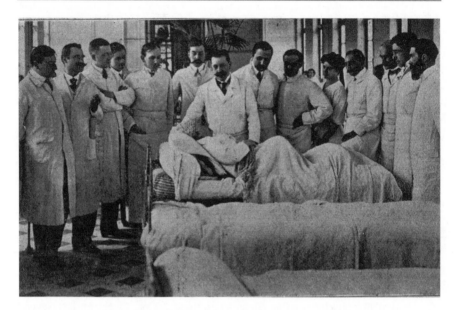

Fig. 8.2 Dr. Jacob Gershberg presenting grand rounds at beside c. 1920. National Library of Medicine

audience and briefly highlight the reason the chosen case is significant. This should be followed by a succinct review of the elements that capture the complexities of the case and a discussion of what reasonable outcomes could have been anticipated, with caveats describing what may have interfered. When presenting to a non-mental health audience, one should understand the basic knowledge the audience has as well as their style in conceptualizing cases.

Anatomy of a Grand Rounds Presentation

While there is certainly no single correct way to present a grand rounds, we would suggest including several elements. First, a discussion of the clinical problem or with regard to background, prevalence, and public-health significance (Copeland et al. 1998). Second, an outline-type figure or slide that can be repeated throughout the presentation to help the audience to reflect on what they've learned, indicate where the presenter will take them next, and encapsulate the general thrust of the talk. Third, slides that take advantage of natural breaks within the grand rounds (e.g., risk factors for the condition, clinical features of the condition, treatment of the condition, complications of treatment, prognostic features of the illness, and predictors or moderators of treatment outcome), summarizing each of these "mini-sections." The less experienced presenter may find it particularly beneficial to rehearse prior to the formal presentation. This will not only decrease presentation-related anxiety, it will help identify points of confusion and may prevent technical difficulties related to the audio-visual material. It is also beneficial to review the presentation with a senior colleague, so as to pinpoint material that may not be received well by the audience (e.g., a term that may be perceived as pejorative, case discussion that may be culturally insensitive).

Presentations at National Conferences

When preparing a presentation for a national conference, it is critical to be familiar with the myriad formats offered. The American Psychiatric Association (APA) has several presentation formats: case conferences, focus live, lectures, forums, seminars, small interactive sessions, symposia, and workshops of different lengths for case presentations. Similarly, the American Academy of Child and Adolescent Psychiatry (AACAP) also offers different programs: clinical case conference, clinical consultation breakfasts, clinical perspectives, and institutes, each of which has a unique format and purpose-specific time allotments. For the psychiatrist or child and adolescent psychiatrist wishing to present at a national conference, the organization (i.e., AACAP, APA, etc.) may provide assistance in determining which format would be most appropriate for the material. Additionally, a presenter may wish to involve colleagues as co-presenters in a program, with agreement as to who is best suited to be the presenter and who the discussant. The role of the discussant is best delegated to a senior colleague with experience in fostering interaction and discussion between the audience and the presenters.

8.2   Preparation for Presentations

Preparing for presentations requires time and organization and does not come easily for many clinicians. For some, giving a presentation will be exciting and provide the opportunity to share clinical material of great interest to them. For others, the endeavor may be associated with anxiety about public speaking and self-doubt. As described in Chap. 3, innate temperament traits dramatically influence an individual's approach to a presentation. Regardless, organization of the material is paramount, whether one is preparing for a symposium at a national meeting or for bedside teaching rounds. With regard to the latter situation, a traditional approach is often utilized. Typically, the organizational tack starts with the patient's chief complaint, history of present illness, past medical and past surgical history, medications, allergies, family history, and the social history (with special attention to early developmental experiences, academics, occupational experience, peer and family relationships). Thereafter, the relevant aspects of the physical and or mental status examination are presented, followed by laboratory findings and neuroimaging studies. Thus, the presenter will typically share a diagnostic impression and proceed to discuss treatment aspects.

After the presentation has been written and "polished," rehearsal, ideally with a colleague serving as the audience, will ensure that it can be delivered within the allotted time. The colleague also may have experience with a particular audience type and be able to help tailor the presentation toward that audience. It is important to acknowledge the role of anxiety in preparing and presenting material. We have seen colleagues who read their presentation with limited interaction with the audience and others who decline to present because of clearly unrealistic fears (e.g., feeling they will never be prepared and will never know everything about the topic). We would remind these colleagues that the goal of a successful presentation is not to present all that is known about a topic but rather to share what one knows about our case or cases, reasons for our interventions, etc.

Confidentiality in Presentations

When considering the educational value of a clinical case presentation or a clinical vignette within a larger presentation, a balance must be struck between "the needs of the profession and the privacy of the patient," though as Gabbard and Williams (2001) point out, "[T]here is no perfect solution to this dilemma." In the psychopharmacologically focused presentations, little demographic or identifying information is provided, and the emphasis is on general symptoms and perhaps laboratory abnormalities. In contrast, the presentation of the "difficult patient or consultation" involves the discussion of critical family conflicts, disagreements with the treatment team, and the personality pathology, all of which may lead to the unintended disclosure of the patient's identity. Thus, it is generally necessary to disguise identifying details, while at the same time maintaining the verisimilitude of the case (Clifft 1986; Tuckett 2000; Gabbard 2000). For these presentations, pseudonyms are often used—as has been the case in this book—and initials are avoided as they can lead the presenter to unknowingly reveal the name of the patient. In some cases, the patient's gender or number of siblings may be changed, and details are omitted unless they are crucial to understanding the patient—though in modifying these superficial details, authors must be careful as the "disguise [may] lead to misleading information about a clinical entity" (Gabbard and Williams 2001). Additionally, it may be important to protect the anonymity of the treatment team. This can be done by modifying the treatment team's specialty, its composition, and the gender or age of its members. When these changes take place, they should be disclosed, to avoid having the audience attempt to "figure out" which patient or treatment team is being presented.

Another approach that is commonly employed to protect anonymity and confidentiality in teaching settings, and that we have used for some of the cases presented herein, is the "composite patient." This involves creating a "fictional" patient using aspects of several prior patients who have been clinically encountered by the presenter (Gabbard and Williams 2001; Blechner 2012).

In our multimedia-friendly information era, grand rounds as well as clinical presentations at meetings and national symposia are frequently audio or video recorded and may be broadcast. In general, arrangements regarding recording are made between the sponsor and the speaker prior to the presentation. At this time the presenter may discuss concerns related to subsequent dissemination of the material with regard to maintaining patient confidentiality. Certainly, if material is to be recorded, one should consider the possibility that it could be viewed at some point by the patient or the family members.

Visual Materials

Visual materials are usually in the form of Powerpoint® and may include embedded video or audio clips. Powerpoint® slides should be easy to read as they lose their usefulness if too crowded with data in small font. The color scheme is particularly important, and light text on a light background or dark text on a dark background should be avoided. A *sans serif* font is generally preferred for readability, and the use of bullet points is helpful highlighting the main points of the slide. Handouts regarding things to be considered in addition to what is being presented can add to a presentation. These handouts can also be copies of the slides. To safeguard confidentiality, however, clinical material should not be included in handouts.

Difficult Situations During Formal Presentations

From time to time, tensions arise between an audience member and the speaker, though this more often occurs during the question-and-answer section of the presentation rather than during the presentation proper. If a presentation involves a difficult psychiatric consultation, the likelihood of presenter/audience-member tensions and conflict is heightened, as formulations are dependent on understanding the parties discussed, patient, family and treatment team, *from the inside out*, which may not be popular with all. Certainly, the etiology of such conflicts are likely multifactorial, and as discussed in this book, differences in temperament, attachment styles, and implicit relational knowing will likely underlie any particular audience member's ability to accept (or not) and to understand (or not) the approach, diagnosis, and treatment described in a given clinical presentation. It is important for the presenter to resist seeing the challenge as a personal affront and to understand that not all audience members will be enamored of the formulations and recommendations presented. Though such disagreements are rarely personal, they may still be somewhat injurious to the presenter and are worthy of further discussion, particularly regarding practical approaches to such a conflict.

The Audience Member Who Monopolizes

Many times we have observed audience members who interject throughout the presentation with their own case examples and approaches to treatment, as well as their version of "clinical pearls"—or who monopolize the question-and-answer session. Not only is this unsettling for the novice presenter but also it interferes with the general learning goals of the presentation. In responding to these repeated interjections and the audience member's sharing of pseudo-expertise, the presenter may first acknowledge their comment as useful (see joining in Chap. 4). In doing so, the presenter will diffuse any immediate conflict, if it exists. Thereafter, the presenter may try a "one-down approach," openly acknowledging and accepting the limitations of presented perspective in the context of larger clinical issues. For example, if an audience member disagrees with the presenter regarding the specific psychotherapeutic approach for major depressive disorder, the presenter might note: "I can see a number of situations in which the treatment that you recommend [dialectical behavioral therapy] would be very helpful to a patient (joining, see Chap. 4). Certainly, my presentation focuses on one small and different aspect of psychotherapy for the depressed patient, and I realize that I will invariably omit other important psychotherapeutic modalities (see reframing, Chap. 4), though I would like to finish my presentation and hope that we can follow up on your comments later today."

The Audience Member Who Attempts to Argue

There will doubtless be times when the presenter has to address an audience member who uses the open forum to strongly state their disagreement to the clinical approach or to suggestions made in the presentation. As with the patient with a difficult temperament style and poor cognitive flexibility (Chap. 3), the presenter should understand that the audience member likely feels personally dismissed and is seeking recognition, either by disagreeing with material or by showing his or her superior knowledge or dislike for the speaker's personality. Obviously, in the course of a discussion or presentation, there will not be enough time to tease apart these aspects of the conflict, and it is thus preferable to acknowledge the audience member's points and, most importantly, to remain calm and confident, which will earn the respect of the audience. It is useful to promptly answer the question, if one was asked, and suggest a one-to-one discussion at the end of the presentation. This will allow dissenter to feel acknowledged, and the presenter can move on to other questions by the audience.

References

Altman LK (2006) Socratic dialogue gives way to powerpoint®. New York Times, 12 Dec 2006
Blechner MJ (2012) Confidentiality: against disguise, for consent. Psychotherapy (Chic) 49 (1):16–18
Clifft MA (1986) Writing about psychiatric patients. Guidelines for disguising case material. Bull Menninger Clin 50(6):511–524
Copeland HL, Hewson MG, Stoller JK et al (1998) Making the continuing medical education lecture effective. J Contin Educ Health Prof 18:227–234
Gabbard GO (2000) Disguise or consent: problems and recommendations concerning the publication and presentation of clinical material. Int J Psychoanal 81:1071–1086
Gabbard GO, Williams P (2001) Preserving confidentiality in writing of case reports. Int J Psychoanal 82:1067–1068
Hull AL, Cullen RJ, Hekelman FP (1989) A retrospective analysis of grand rounds in continuing medical education. J Contin Educ Health Prof 9(4):257–266

Lorin MI, Palazzi DL, Turner TL et al (2008) What is a clinical pearl and what is its role in medical education? Med Teach 30(9–10):870–874

Sackett DL, Rosenberg WM, Gray JA et al (1996) Evidence based medicine: what it is and what it isn't. Br Med J 312:71–72

Tuckett D (2000) Reporting clinical events in the journal: towards the constructing of a special case. Int J Psychoanal 81:1065–1069

Index

A

Abuse, 14
Academic hospitals, 126
Academic medical centers, 3
Acculturation, 6
Ackerman, N.W., 66
Activity level, 48
Adolescents, 37, 43, 44, 51
Advanced-practice nurses, 96
Afifi, W.A., 70
African Americans, 131
Ainsworth, M.D., 24, 26, 28
Akhtar, S., 17
Alexander, F., 28
Allen, J.G., 23, 33
Altarac, M., 40
Alternative medicine, 132
Altman, L.K., 139
Ambivalence, 97, 104, 105, 107
American Academy of Child and Adolescent
    Psychiatry (AACAP), 85, 86, 141
American Academy of Child and Adolescent
    Psychiatry, Bill of Rights, 85, 86
American Hospital Association, 96
American Psychiatric Association, 115, 141
American Psychiatric Association 2000, 22
American Psychiatric Association 2013, 2,
    4, 37
Anal, 11
Anesthesiologist, 96
Anger, 74, 76, 79, 89, 130
Anonymity, 142
Anxiety, 38, 40, 44, 45, 50, 51, 53, 55, 68, 75,
    78, 84, 90, 91, 97, 100, 103, 106, 109,
    110, 125, 128, 131, 133, 140–142
Anxious attachment, 24
Appelbaum, P.S., 118
Aron, L., 9, 30
Arras, J.D., 113, 120

Ascherman, L.I., 113, 120
Asthma, 79
Attachment, 125, 126, 130
    style, 51–53, 57, 61, 69, 74, 76, 82, 91, 96,
        97, 100, 102, 109
    theory, 24, 27, 87
Audience, 137, 139–144
    members, 139, 143
Autonomy, 61, 62, 106, 109, 113, 115, 116,
    119, 120
Avoidant attachment, 24

B

Barker, P., 66
Bateman A, 23
Beckman, H.B., 5
Beneficence, 62, 109, 113, 116, 119, 120
Benoit, D., 24
Bereavement, 40, 88, 89
Bernheim, S.M., 129
Berry, L.L., 110
Bion, W., 109
Bio-psycho-social, 2–4
Birch, H.G., 47
Bisexual, 132
Black, M.J., 12
Blackwell, K.A., 42
Blechner, M.J., 142
Bleiberg, E., 43
Borderline, 17, 23, 25
Boston Process and Change Study Group, 29
Bowen, M., 66
Bowlby, J., 24, 25, 28, 29, 46, 66
Brenner, C., 12
Bretherton, I., 27
Brody, G.H., 87
Bromberg, P., 30
Bronheim, H.E., 3

S.V. Delgado and J.R. Strawn, *Difficult Psychiatric Consultations*,
DOI 10.1007/978-3-642-39552-9, © Springer-Verlag Berlin Heidelberg 2014